What people are saying . . .

"Mary Lou Falcone's matchless gift for conveying the voices and artistry of others has taken her to the pinnacle of success in classical music public relations. In her powerful memoir, *I Didn't See It Coming*, she finally employs that talent to tell her own story, entering into the perspectives of those closest to her at pivotal moments in her life. It is a fascinating approach, made more moving by the inclusion of poetry, the illustrations of her beloved husband, and her own unflinching journal of his final illness. Beyond being essential reading for those caring for someone with Lewy body dementia (LBD), *I Didn't See It Coming* is a beautifully rendered, inspiring chronicle of determination, resilience, and boundless love."

—RENÉE FLEMING, Soprano

"A beautiful story of music, faith, compassion, friendship, and undying love."

—DAVID HYDE PIERCE, Actor

"Mary Lou Falcone has written a compelling memoir that guides the reader with drama, empathy, humor, and vision through her remarkable life, punctuated by the continuing saga of her great love for her husband and soulmate, Nicky Zann. During this voyage, we meet great artists, international personalities, and her many remarkable friends and family. This volume is a must-read for anyone who has had to deal with the debilitating and tragic results of Lewy body dementia, here seen through the detailed and arduous challenges involving Nicky's battle with this nefarious disease."

—JOSEPH W. POLISI, President Emeritus, The Juilliard School

"Witnessing my dear friend ML turn her personal story of love and loss into a universal one of commitment to caregiving and a mission to help others understand the mysteries of often-camouflaged Lewy body dementia has been a revelation to me, as well as a generous gift to anyone who reads *I Didn't See It Coming.*"

—**MARY BETH PEIL**, Friend and Actor

"Mary Lou Falcone writes like no other about Lewy body dementia. With love, insight, and compassion, she shares that during extremely difficult moments strength kicks in and a painful journey can also be one from which you can emerge with a new sense of purpose. An important book for caregivers who are struggling with someone affected by dementia, especially LBD."

—**JAAP VAN ZWEDEN**, Music Director, New York Philharmonic
—**AALTJE VAN ZWEDEN**, Author and Founder,
Papageno Foundation

"Finally, Lewy body dementia—a disease that has been vastly unknown and misunderstood for decades—comes out of the shadows. Mary Lou Falcone's candid and intriguing memoir enlightens us on the disease and the difficulties of caregiving, while inspiring us with a life well-lived and filled with love."

—**NORMA LOEB**, Founder, Lewy Body Dementia Resource Center

I DIDN'T SEE IT COMING

SCENES OF LOVE, LOSS, AND
LEWY BODY DEMENTIA

MARY LOU FALCONE

WITH ILLUSTRATIONS BY
NICKY ZANN

EAST END PRESS
NEW YORK • BRIDGEHAMPTON

A portion of the proceeds from the sale of this book will be donated to the *Lewy Body Dementia Resource Center*

Published by
EAST END PRESS
Bridgehampton, NY

ISBN: 978173452689-9
Ebook ISBN: 979898732660-2

First Edition

Book Design by Pauline Neuwirth, Neuwirth & Associates, Inc.
Cover Design by David Fassett

Manufactured in the United States of America
10 9 8 7 6 5 4 3 2 1

For Nicky,
my soulmate for eternity

Contents

PART SEVEN

2019 & 2020
THE LAST JOURNEY

APPENDICES

HELP AND RESOURCES FOR LEWY BODY
AND RELATED DEMENTIA

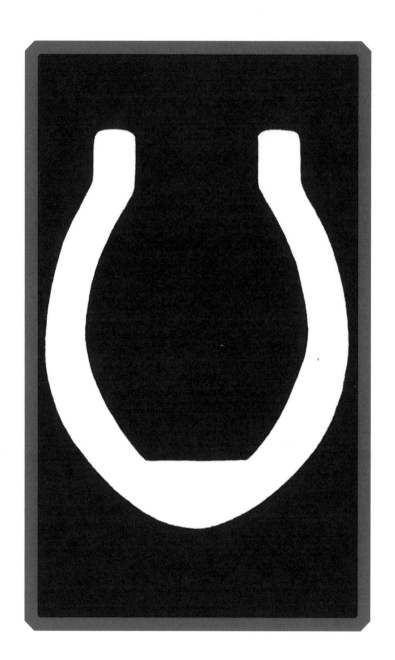

Author's Note

I am grateful to so many who patiently listened and followed my odyssey to bring this book to life. While navigating some painful moments of grieving, this cathartic journey turned out to be full of hope and joy. I allowed myself to feel it all, the love and the loss, and to relive it, emerging with a new sense of purpose.

The thank-you list starts with my mother, Mary DeStefano Falcone, my father, Louis V. Falcone, and my grandfather, Dominick DeStefano—the anchors of my life. My soulmate, Nicholas "Nicky" Zann, also referred to throughout as NZ, was not only the love of my life but the inspiration and catalyst for this book. Shortly before he passed away, he encouraged me to write, and I could feel him sitting on my shoulder through the whole process, shining his light and wisdom on my path.

When I read my earliest attempts aloud to my brother, Louis J. Falcone, and my sister, Angela Falcone DePalma, they urged me to go deeper, to excavate my primal, early emotions. They generously shared their stories and opinions about growing up and gave me permission to use it all—an act of love.

Upon completing a first draft, I shared it with a trio of trusted friends: Mary Beth Peil, Véronique Firkusny, and my sister, Angel, all avid readers with disparate points of view. Interestingly, they too pushed for more transparency, encouragingly and critically cheering me on throughout numerous rewrites. Others who offered invaluable information and perspectives include Katrine

Ames, Lisa Bellamore, Dr. Jason A. Cohen, Margaret Crane, Denise Dailey, Stephanie DePalma, Judith Frankfurt, Cathy Mackell Frantz, Diane DeStefano Giovanniello, Laney Gradus, Gwyneth Kirkbride, Rick Kot, Judith Kurnick, Ellyn Kusmin, Eriq La Salle, Norma Loeb, Dr. Leon Meytin, James Oestreich, David Hyde Pierce, Jane Scovell, Aaltje and Jaap van Zweden, Elizabeth Vecchione, Christine von der Linn, Ruthie DeStefano West, and Kathryn Yatrakis.

A stroke of good fortune came my way through my dear friend and colleague Philippa Polskin, when she introduced me to Holly Peppe, an extraordinary and brilliant woman who became my first editor. Holly taught me so much, helping me to optimize my narrative by probing, shaping, pushing, and polishing, all the while being a kind, honest, and perfect taskmaster. I was so lucky to have been taken under her thoughtful and capable wing.

With insight and wisdom, East End Press publisher Pauline Neuwirth, who understood my mission, encouraged me to explore more deeply the difficult, dark days of Lewy body dementia, especially the final two years of Nicky's life. She introduced me to my second editor, Kathleen Doherty, whose experience, sagacity, and laser-sharp literary skills propelled me to tackle the major hurdle I had been avoiding—the daunting last rewrite to ultimately reveal deeply buried emotions in order to tell a more personal and poignant story.

My story is full of extraordinary people to whom I am grateful. They include my family, both immediate and extended, plus John Binsfeld, Grace Bumbry, Dr. John Cahill, Rildia Bee O'Bryan Cliburn, Van Cliburn, Andrew Corsaro, Bonnie Lueders Corsaro, Frank Corsaro, Rosamond Cross, Avery Fisher, Renée Fleming, Dorothy Fulmer, Eufemia Giannini Gregory, Lee Hoiby, Bob Holton, Vincent Ioppolo, Silva Khundiashvili, Leroy Lenox, Amanda Leone, Andrew Leone, Rhoda Levine, Norma Loeb,

Riccardo Muti, Mary Beth Peil, Joseph W. Polisi, Mary Jo Quay, Gus Rego, Nadja Salerno-Sonnenberg, George Schaefer, Robert Shaw, Marcia Sketchley, Vladimir Sokoloff, Alexander Toradze, Alix Williamson, Lanford Wilson, Efrem Zimbalist Sr.—and a few others who shall remain anonymous.

PART ONE

The Arc of
Shaping a Life

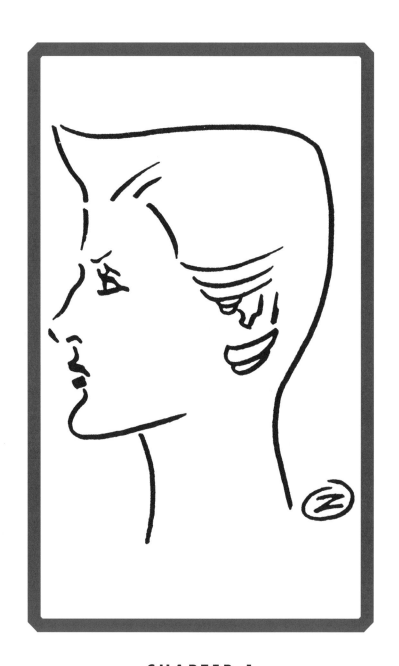

CHAPTER 1

So, Why Now?

Over the years, whenever I was asked, "When are you going to write your book," I would quickly reply, "Never!" Lesson learned: Never say never.

So, why have I reversed my emphatic, lifelong resolve? The simple answer: The arc of life has taken some dramatic turns that I didn't see coming, and my heart tells me it's time to share.

My life path was charted when I was ten years old. With a cruel stroke of fate, my father was robbed of his ability to speak and needed constant care. Being the eldest child and forced to embrace responsibility earlier than most, I built emotional walls to protect myself from feeling helpless and overwhelmed. I didn't dare indulge in feelings, because getting through the day would have been too difficult.

But my life changed when, through music, I discovered my God-given gift—a talent for singing and performing that enabled me to safely express my emotions. My ten-year-old self suddenly felt free to create, to build, to dream. Still, seeing my father incapacitated from his stroke and unable to support us, I understood the necessity and power of both communication and caregiving, which would eventually become the leitmotifs of my life. Singing was to be my point of entry, an opening to a world I never before could have imagined.

For decades I have shied away from the words *I, me,* and *my,* preferring to focus on the lives and careers of others, often writing in their voices through my work in public relations. So, why now, after so many years of privacy and choosing to stay behind the scenes, would I publicly share my story? The experience of caregiving—first for my father and more recently for my beloved late husband, Nicholas "Nicky" Zann, as he struggled with Lewy body dementia—was life-altering and life-affirming. In telling my story, I hope the words, especially those about LBD, will resonate with others, offering information and affirmation along with hope during times of overwhelming stress.

Because I have spent a lifetime consciously deflecting negativity and redirecting everything toward the positive, this story is a tribute to love and resilience. It's an homage to Nicky as well as to the other voices you will hear throughout—both personal and professional—all of whom had a major influence on my life. Some were sources of wisdom, guidance, comfort, and challenge, while others offered cautionary tales of insight. All were vital to shaping who I am today.

Early on in the writing process, I decided to use Nicky's brilliant illustrations from his best-selling, fortune-telling game, *The Answer Deck,* to advance each chapter. We had always wanted to collaborate on a book, and now we have. With these special drawings and the spirit of Nicky by my side, I felt the mosaic of our lives come together as I wrote. Once again, the universe offered the gift.

When I began the process, this narrative was solely in my voice. As I revisited years of memories, many seminal characters from the past spoke to me so directly that I felt compelled to speak through their voices, the experiences being as much theirs as mine.

In the end, I hope the journey that emerges will inspire, inform, amuse, and at times offer solace to the readers who choose to come along.

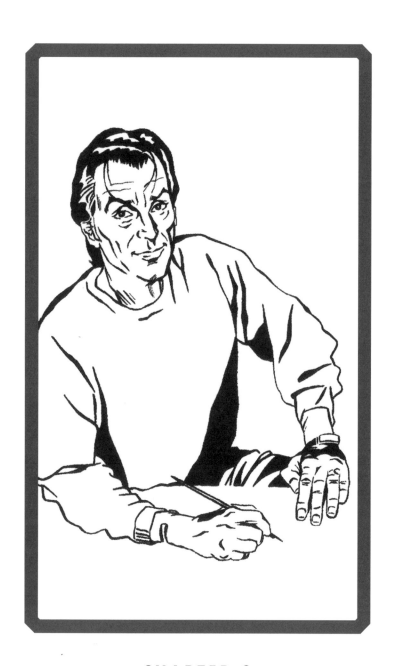

CHAPTER 2

Nicky

My heart will always belong to Nicky.

Nicholas T. Zann, known to all as *Nicky* and to many as *Uncle Nicky*, was a force to be reckoned with from the day he came into the world—June 7, 1943.

One of my favorite descriptions of Nicky comes from dear friends who eulogized him in *The New York Times* as "unique, original, ever generous, and unforgettable." Yes, he was a one-of-a-kind, never to be forgotten, force of nature.

Nicky's childhood in the 1940s and '50s set the tone for his life, a life that was anything but ordinary. Soon after his birth in New York City, he was whisked off, wrapped in a pink blanket (it was wartime and blue blankets were in short supply), to spend his earliest years in Lakeland, Florida, and Biloxi, Mississippi, where his father was in Air Force pilot training during World War II. When Nicky was five, the family returned East, this time settling in Little Neck, Long Island.

Showing early signs of both musical and artistic talent, Nicky was lucky to have parents who happily noticed and nurtured both.

His mother, Ellen, a homemaker of French, Greek, and Irish descent, understood artists. She grew up with a musician father, Nick Michaelis, who had done everything from washing dishes for the privilege of playing cornett in the Boston Symphony before the turn of the last century, to finally making a decent living as a musician by joining Buffalo Bill's Wild West show around 1900. Grandfather Nick would also become a sideman for Jimmie Rodgers, widely known as "the Father of Country Music." Grandson Nicky clearly inherited the musical gene.

Nicky's father Ernest, also first-generation Greek and French, started as a Western Union delivery boy in his youth before going on to become a banker-turned-certified-public-accountant. Being a perspicacious father, he recognized his son's free spirit. Together, the Zanns were parents of remarkable insight when it came to raising their gifted and strong-willed child.

As the eldest, with two younger sisters, Nicky forged a unique path. In grade school, he won drawing contests, giving him scholarships and entrée to Rhodes, a New York City private school that clearly didn't suit him. He was mischievous and, at age ten, more interested in singing in a gospel quartet, the Aladdins. Nicky sang lead and was joined by a set of musical twins and a talented young black lad; he loved every minute of after-school rehearsals and performances with his buddies. Along the way, at age thirteen, on a train ride from New York City to his Little Neck home, he had a chance meeting with his idol, Rudi Maugeri, founder of the Crew-Cuts, the famed 1950s doo-wop vocal quartet. Evidently not long after this encounter, Rudi was unexpectedly introduced to Nicky's mother at a Little Neck cocktail party, and connecting the dots he quipped: "So, Nicky's your son? Your kid knows more about me than I know about myself."

Laughing, because she knew exactly how obsessed her son was, Ellen Zann told Maugeri that Nicky was a budding performer who wanted to be just like the Crew-Cuts.

Showing interest, Rudi asked, "Where is he performing these days?" As fate would have it, that very evening Nicky was performing at the nearby Hotel James, actually a *hôtel de passe* (commonly known as a bordello) in Great Neck's Spinney Hill section.

Rudi went to hear him and immediately said, "Kid, I want you to sing for my manager, George Brown."

An audition was quickly arranged, and George, who happened to be of Greek heritage, took a shine to the "young Greek kid," believed in his talent, and signed him up on the spot. What is so incredible about this stroke of fate is that George Brown not only managed the Crew-Cuts but had been Tony Bennett's first manager as well. Now in the big leagues, Nicky, much to his chagrin, was often referred to as the "baby Elvis."

So, by age fourteen, the professionally managed Nicky was playing the local honkytonks and buckets of blood (as he called them), often performing behind chicken wire, which protected him from flying beer bottles when things got wild. During those days, which were anything but glamorous, he often played on the same shows as Connie Francis, Patsy Cline, Johnny Cash, Jackie Wilson, and Jerry Lee Lewis, with his parents' blessing. Truth be told, I think they wisely knew that Nicky couldn't be stopped and prayed he would stay out of harm's way. Miraculously, he escaped the drug scene (he had no interest in it, not even in experimenting), but he did love his nightly rum and Coke . . . to soothe his throat or so he claimed.

While being managed by George Brown, Nicky actually turned down the opportunity to record "Itsy Bitsy Teeny Weeny Yellow Polka Dot Bikini," saying, "Georgie, I know it's going to be a hit, but I'm not the right person to sing it. It doesn't evoke what I'm all about."

George is said to have responded, "Baby, evoke? What? Just tell me one thing, what do you have against eating?"

Nicky did go on to have a hit for Roulette Records with "Southern Belle," the popularity of which was boosted throughout the country when he performed it on Dick Clark's popular television program *American Bandstand*.

By age sixteen, Nicky, who fronted as his band's lead singer and often played piano for the songs he composed, switched to the nationally known promoter Troy Stevens, one of the leading black managers of his day, who better understood Nicky's music and went on the road with him and his seasoned band, The Vitamins. Touring extensively in the South, Northeast, Texas, and Canada, and now a teen idol frequently featured in fanzines and magazines for teens, Nicky was appearing on the same bills as The Cadillacs, The Temptations, Little Anthony and the Imperials, Dale Hawkins, and Pat Boone. Nicky Zann and The Vitamins were even featured playing the music of Tom O'Horgan for underground films written and directed by Robert Downey Sr. It is interesting to note that, until the day Georgie died, Nicky and George Brown remained close friends. And when the teenaged Nicky asked Georgie to tear up his contract, George not only agreed but actually threw it into the roaring fire in his office. George understood that Nicky needed more than he was willing or able to do at the time.

The rock 'n' roll era for Nicky lasted a little more than seven years, making his attendance at Manhattan's High School of Art and Design in the late 1950s and early '60s a challenge. His performance schedule, coupled with carousing in the after-hours clubs, made getting up most mornings nearly impossible. And while he often skipped classes or slept through the ones he did attend, he managed to graduate with flying colors.

Throughout these performing years, art remained his passion. From age ten, Nicky was determined to meet his cartooning hero, Alfred Andriola, creator of the syndicated *Kerry Drake* comic strip. Obsessed with Andriola's work, on a whim he wrote to Alfred who invited Nicky to visit his Greenwich Village townhouse studio.

When this long-haired, skinny kid with good manners (Alfred often commented on this) appeared on Alfred's doorstep, a lifelong mentorship and friendship began. Alfred became Nicky's artistic father. Nicky often said that being around Alfred and his partner, Rick DiCecca, was like growing up in a real-life version of *La Cage aux Folles*. In the world of comics, Nicky went on to draw *Batman* for DC Comics; and for Charlton Comics, he created "Love Comic," a new style of comic that was to become famous, eventually finding a home in the Victoria and Albert Museum.

Nicky's last official performance as a rock 'n' roller was in 1965, when, by popular GI demand, he was invited to perform at the prestigious Lufthansa Airlines Ball in Frankfurt, Germany. Using his earnings, a princely sum of $5,000 for singing two songs, he and his new, twenty-year-old wife spent a full year touring Europe.

When Nicky returned to the States, the twenty-two-year-old knew that art was his real calling. Even though he loved rock 'n' roll and was flattered that Bobby Darin and Terry Melcher were still hoping to manage him, Nicky was resolute—his rock 'n' roll days were over. He enrolled in New York's School of Visual Arts, where he became the protégé of Burne Hogarth, well-known *Tarzan* illustrator, and Jack Potter.

Unfortunately, Nicky's young bride was counting on being a rock star's wife, not the wife of a struggling artist, and so, the marriage of less than two years was annulled. At Visual Arts, Nicky met and married a fellow student, the extremely talented and beautiful Mary Jo Quay, and this marriage was to last for fifteen years.

Nicky's art career grew quickly and became legendary. In addition to paintings displayed in private collections, such as the Curtis Institute in Philadelphia, his "Love Comic" art, as mentioned, hangs in the permanent pop art collection of London's Victoria and Albert Museum. Several of the "Love Comic" pieces from that collection were borrowed in 2016 by the TextielMuseum of the Netherlands for its exhibition *Pop Art Fabrics & Fashion—From Warhol to Westwood (1956–1976)*. The TextielMuseum alleged that "[Roy] Lichtenstein used the comics and cartoons of this acclaimed graphic designer [Nicky Zann] as the main inspiration for his art."

My brother, Louis, a fellow artist, described Nicky's work best in a condolence letter when he wrote: "Nicky's talents and knowledge slowly unfolded to me over the years. It took me some years to fully appreciate this complex, sort of brilliant, crazy guy. He was often over the top but always cleverly funny with a touch of evil genius. His stories often took us on a winding journey . . . . He had a full and colorful life to draw from. Yes he loved to be the jokester, but there was knowledge and understanding of how the world works and its history, that most of us never retained. The world according to Uncle Nicky through his teenage rock 'n' roll to his amazing caricatures and cartoons, along with being a force in the art world as an illustrator/painter made him quite the renaissance man with a huge heart. Uncle Nicky was a success in any form you could imagine."

I mention all of this specifically to point out that Nicky never bragged about any of this and rarely talked about the celebrated achievements of his fifty years in the art world. His body of work included everything from Broadway posters, book and magazine covers, comic books, and illustrations for advertising campaigns to caricatures and oil paintings. Add to this creative projects like his best-selling Running Press fortune-telling game, *The Answer Deck*, and throw in a successful line of beaded couture dresses featuring his humorous drawings. Well, you get the picture, a nonending stream of creativity exhibiting the breadth and depth of his legacy. However, even with all of this to his credit, Nicky would much rather regale you with stories about the early days of rock 'n' roll, often going to the piano to demonstrate. The rocker never completely left the building . . .

In later years, Nicky's work was auctioned, and posthumously still is, by Swann Auction Galleries. Swann's former Illustration Art Specialist Christine von der Linn remembers Nicky as a person "gifted with a talented hand and blessed with a beautiful soul and lightning-quick wit that always showed in his work." She continued: "We at Swann were excited to offer Nicky's work because of its skill and energy. Every work was tinged with his keen wit. It was always great fun to walk through exhibitions with Nicky, who delighted in seeing his own work hung in the company of such illustration icons as Charles Addams, Ludwig Bemelmans, and Edward Gorey. Watching his enthusiastic reactions to the various works and hearing his take on them, sometimes treating us to background art world trivia and insights, allowed us to see our own offerings in a new light."

Nicky had the distinct ability to make everyone he encountered feel special, treating all with respect, dignity, and equality—from busboys in restaurants, all of whose names he made a point of knowing, to heads of state. It was a one-size-fits-all treatment.

He was proud of his Greek and Irish roots, but especially loved his French heritage and spoke the language fluently, if a bit archaically according to our French friends.

Nicky loved life, loved God, was deeply spiritual, and believed in the power of prayer. He had a kind word for everyone and never said anything he didn't mean.

We met in 1973, became a couple in 1983, married in 2017, and, in Nicky's words, "had a great run together." Until . . . I had to say goodbye.

Special moments continue to surface—like the first glimpse of the sun as it comes over the ocean on a beautiful summer morning, the fresh smell of earth after a spring rain, the vibrancy of autumn colors, the quiet starkness of the first winter snow, the joyous sound of children's laughter—they all remind me of Nicky.

CHAPTER 3

I Say Goodbye . . .

Nicky," I say, "it's just the two of us," as it has been for months. June 7, 2020, we celebrate your seventy-seventh birthday with good wishes pouring in from all over the world. How loved you are. As beautiful as this is, it takes so much energy out of you that the next day you are fragile and exhausted and sleep for hours.

Your descent has begun. This devastating, progressive disease, Lewy body dementia, is stealing you away, taking a little more from you each day.

It's time for the "chair with wheels," which you accept only because I tell you it's a gift from our treasured doctor whom you call "the angel." This slight deception serves its purpose. Days are spent in total repose with an occasional outing down to the Hudson River, aided of course by "the chair." Oh, how you love the air, the wind on your face, the sunshine—yes, even you, who always loved gray, gloomy days, now prefer the sunshine.

You don't totally understand COVID-19—who among us does?—and the restrictions annoy you.

Food has no appeal. Wine has no appeal.

You don't always know who I am, but you are comforted by my touch, the sound of my voice.

You have stopped saying, "I will beat this."

Your "angel" doctor makes a house call, hiding his shock at how quickly you are declining.

Toward the end of June, sensing the end is near, I pull out your ingenious fortune-telling card game, *The Answer Deck*, the one you created and designed many years ago. I have always believed in its power, and now I put it to the acid test, asking where you will be by the end of July 2020. The answer is *home*.

It's now Tuesday, July 7, and your adored three-year-old godson Andrew comes to visit with your niece Amanda. When Andrew, playing a favorite game, calls out, "Hello, pirate Nicky," and gets no response, he just kneels next to your chair and lovingly hugs your knees. He seems to understand your silence and moves aside to play by himself. What extraordinary insight and wisdom from a small child.

You eat two bites of lunch and that's it, you stop eating for good, and I know it's time for hospice.

With hospice in place on Thursday, July 9, I also make sure that arrangements are in place for the end. Your sense of humor flashes before me as I am asked by the funeral director if I prefer a pine or cardboard box for your last trip. Finding the question very funny, I laughingly say, "Pine, of course." I am reminded of a shared memory that always made us laugh—all my mother's canine friends going to the great beyond in cardboard Xerox boxes.

That same day, you stop drinking any liquid. It's time to gather family and friends to say goodbye. You insist upon getting up and being wheeled into our living room to be part of the gathering, and nothing will stop you from being the host. You so sweetly acknowledge everyone in the room: my family, your family, our loving friends.

On Saturday, July 11, we are alone again. Now you are free to just be, no longer needing to be the entertainer. I shower you that morning, knowing how you love to be clean and fresh. God must have given me an extra surge of strength, because mercifully at 5:00 a.m., I could carry you to the shower without dropping you.

Later that morning, I call my lifelong friend Mary Beth Peil (MB). She arrives and stays for the next three days and nights, sleeping on the living room couch, always with an ear to what might be needed—a gift to us both.

I must figure out a way to get you last rites, and I am now more determined than ever, though no priest will enter our apartment during COVID. I call upon a priest acquaintance, Father John, and ask if he has ever done last rites via speakerphone.

His answer is, "No, but why not?" And so, we proceed, and he empowers me at the end of the call to administer the sign of the cross on your palms and forehead with lavender oil to complete the sacrament. You, my love, are blessed and in a state of grace, and I am relieved.

On Sunday and Monday, you still insist on trying to get out of bed to use the bathroom—and with help, at least on Sunday, you succeed.

By Monday night, you are closing down. I sleep right next to you as I always have, now listening to the changing patterns of your breathing, the morphine every few hours easing your journey.

Daylight breaks on Bastille Day, July 14, 2020. You gently pass at 10:20 a.m. The struggle has ended. I study your face, now at peace. I hold your hand and quietly weep tears of sadness that I have lost you, tears of joy that you no longer have to suffer. You are free.

As MB and I prepare you for your final journey, I think about the two Marys—Magdalene and the Virgin—who attended Jesus at the hour of his death. It's a bit irreverent, but knowing your sense of humor, I am sure you would totally appreciate what's coming next as I ask MB which Mary she would prefer to be. Her answer is Magdalene, and I am delighted, as I prefer the other Mary.

And so, the two Marys, Mary Lou and Mary Beth, prepare you for the final journey. We work quickly, making sure you look as you would have wished. Tonsorial splendor is a must for you in death, as it was in life. I have chosen an outfit that is exactly what you would have worn on one of our dates: your navy pin-striped blazer, long-sleeved black T-shirt, black jeans, and loafers, with a silk navy scarf wrapped around your neck and light blue pocket square in your jacket breast pocket. You are fully ready to make your perfect, final exit.

As a candle burns beside you, I spend a private hour with you saying my last goodbye and thanking you for our wonderful life together—promising to always remember your wise and comforting words, "We have had a great run, we cannot be sad." This is now my mantra, thank you.

When the funeral home escorts arrive at 2:00 p.m. sharp to transport you, they comment, "What an elegant gentleman." I smile, knowing how happy this would make you.

As you are leaving our home for the last time, I give you a final kiss at the front door, whispering, "I love you . . . have a safe journey *home*."

Your dignity maintained, you pass on as you lived—with grace and love.

God bless you and rest in peace, my beloved Nicky . . .

PART TWO

1940s, 1950s, 1960s

Family and Early Influential Voices

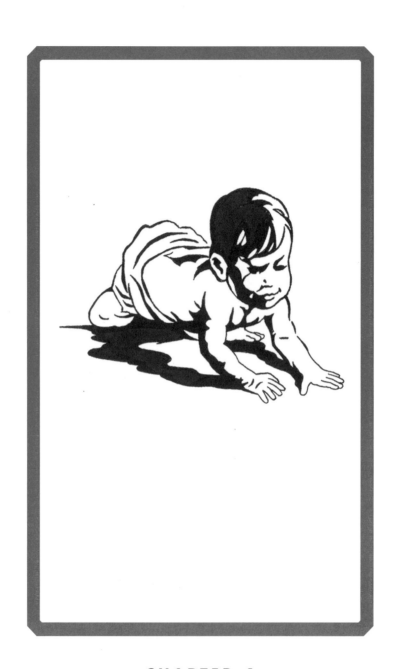

CHAPTER 4

My Story Begins . . .

. . . DECADES BEFORE I KNEW NICKY, WITH MANY influential characters who were essential in shaping my future, paving the way for events and happenings that I didn't see coming.

Childhood scenes fill my memory—some vivid, some hidden until now.

"Why is my baby sister getting all the attention? She's spoiling everything," I tell my favorite toy, Lambie, as I hug him. I tell him everything, we are always together. "You know, my little brother is fun, just like you, Lambie. It's okay if he's here, but I wish she would go away."

Before my sister and brother are born, I have Mommy and Daddy all to myself. I like it that way. Mommy reads to me all the time. I love reciting nursery rhymes—my favorite, of course, "Mary Had a Little Lamb," because my name is Mary Lou. Mommy sometimes takes me with her on the bus, and one day the bus driver says, "What a beautiful little girl, but she'll never be as beautiful as her mother." Mommy laughs, but I know she likes hearing this because she always talks about what he said.

Daddy works hard during the week, and on the weekends, we play. One Saturday, Mommy asks Daddy to take me for a haircut.

He comes home hiding me behind his back. Mommy takes one look and bursts into tears—all my golden curls are gone. Another time Daddy and I go to the playground, and he puts me on a big swing. But I'm only two and a half, and I don't know how to hold on. Flying into the air, I land chin first on a sharp rock. Many stitches and lots of crying later, I calm down, but Mommy is still upset and says to Daddy, "Louie, how could you let this happen?"

I know I am loved, but now everything seems to be all about that new baby. I feel left out, really left out.

Since wetting your pants seems to get attention, I decide at age five, I can do it too. Well, this is a big mistake. Mommy is so mad that she puts a baby diaper on me saying, "If you act like a baby, we'll treat you like a baby." If that isn't bad enough, she insists that I answer the ringing doorbell wearing that stupid baby diaper.

Now I am confused and really mad! I take a metal Band-Aid box and smash Maudie's face—she's my favorite doll, the one with real hair. I guess choosing my doll is better than my baby sister, but Mommy is mad, even madder than I am. Out comes the nasty breadboard. I get really scared when I see it. It's the signal for a big spanking, the bad kind that really hurts—ouch, ouch, and more ouch! I get all the bad spankings. It's not fair.

I love Mommy so much. I love Daddy too, but I want Mommy's attention, and boy, do I get it, breadboard and all. But when I am not doing naughty things, Mommy is very loving.

Mommy brings Maudie to the doll hospital to get her face fixed. I wonder if Mommy loves my brother the most, then my baby sister, then Maudie, and then me. It seems like I always come last. Sometimes I feel so alone.

Thank goodness for Grandpa, who lives with us. With him I come first. He loves me.

Just after my sister is born, we all move from the city to the country. Everyone is happy. We now live on a beautiful street in a house that is all ours, not like the one in the other place where another family had the other half. And we kids have a big backyard to play in.

The new house is very dirty, and Mommy says, "It looks like pigs lived here!" She scrubs for days and makes it all shiny. Hard work is nothing new for Mommy.

Things are good. I feel safe. I have new friends and so does my brother. My sister is still too little for friends, but she has us. Now that I know she's here to stay, I actually think she's sweet.

Most of the time I'm well-behaved, but I have one very bad habit—I talk back a lot, and Mommy and Daddy hate this. Mommy washes my mouth out with soap, hoping that will cure me, and Daddy, using his mad voice (usually he's so calm and nice), says: "One more remark like that from you, young lady, and I will knock your teeth down your throat. Never speak to your mother like that again!" Scary! And while I know he would never hurt me, he always stands up for Mommy, no matter what.

But Grandpa comes to the rescue. It's good he still lives with us. He always makes things better for me. He is my hero. I am his *Dolly.*

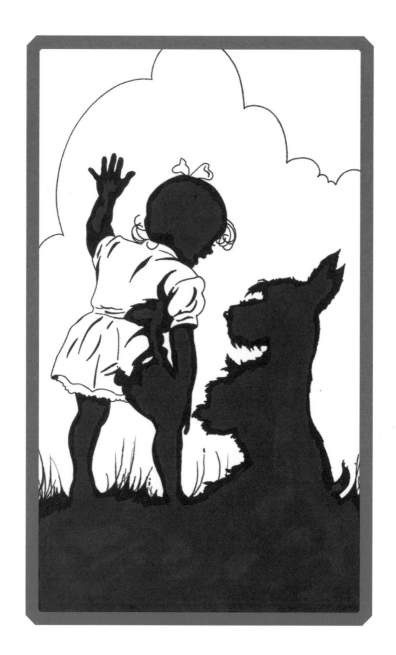

CHAPTER 5

Grandpa

MY HERO WAS GRANDPA, A TALL HANDSOME MAN with sad, blue eyes who spoke only Italian. He was humble and kind and had endured an immigrant's hard life. After his wife tragically died in her twenties, and without any formal education, he managed to raise and care for his four small children. He had many opportunities to remarry. One lady in particular was a grande dame, the mother of New Jersey Mafia boss Angelo "Gyp" DeCarlo. Mrs. DeCarlo adored my grandfather and, in the Roaring Twenties, would pick him up for their dates in her chauffeur-driven limousine.

Even though this marriage prospect would have vastly improved the quality of this hatmaker's daily life, my grandfather always said a polite, "No. I don't want my children to have a stepmother." He was a principled, stubborn, and simple man for whom honesty and dignity were paramount. Determined to make life work on his own humble terms, he shouldered the responsibility for his family alone.

Right to the end of his life, he signed any document requiring his signature with an X. Grandpa died in 1959, when I was fourteen. All his life, he loved his homemade red wine, and even when he was diagnosed with severe diabetes and was told to stop drinking, he continued to enjoy it. He lost a leg to gangrene. He was a fighter, but the diabetes would eventually win. When I went to the hospital to say goodbye, he thought I was my mother and kept saying: "Don't bring Dolly here, I don't want her to see me like this. Please tell her I love her."

In our family, everyone had a champion: My mother's favorite was my brother (the only son in an Italian household generally occupies that place of honor); my father adored my baby sister; and I had Grandpa, my knight in shining armor. To this day, I cannot talk about him without tears welling up. I always felt safe when he was around, he was my protector. *Ti amo sempre*, Grandpa.

call my granddaughter Mary Lou my Dolly. She loves me unconditionally. Since the day she was born, we've had a special bond. Maybe it's because I wasn't allowed to raise her mother that I'm making up for what I missed. When my wife, along with our infant daughter, suddenly died leaving me with our four children, my daughter, Mary, was two years old. The State of New Jersey ordered me to place her in an orphanage: "It isn't proper for a little girl to be raised by a single father in a house full of boys," they said. I hated being forced to leave my baby with strangers, but I didn't know how to fight the authorities. I keep thinking maybe Dolly is my second chance. This time it's different, Dolly cannot be taken away from me.

Mary, my daughter, seems to understand. She welcomes the special connection between her daughter, Mary Lou, and me.

I take Dolly with me to bars where I drink with my friends. She sits on the countertop and sips a soda, just watching as I talk with my cronies. I take her to pet the deer or to see the trains go by, and she watches contentedly.

We often sit in the backyard. She always has time for my stories. I tell her about my adventures in Italy as a guard for King Umberto I and how I helped to save his life from an assassination attempt. This was in the late 1890s, just before I decided to come to America. When I arrived here in 1905, I worked as a hatter, and Dolly loves to play with the hats I made. Since I speak only Italian, I'm never sure if she understands all the words. It really doesn't matter; the words are not what's important.

In the living room, I sit and listen as she plays the piano I bought for her. She sings just for me. I love her, and I love to hear her voice.

A few years later when Dolly is almost ten, her father falls ill and I have to move out. I am told that Dolly sits night after night at the kitchen table, weeping uncontrollably for her grandpa. I weep for her too.

As I prepare to leave this earth, I keep thinking that Dolly is my daughter—and perhaps in a way she is.

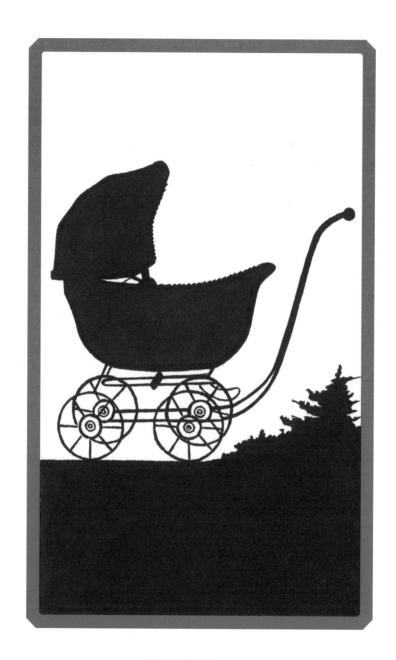

CHAPTER 6

Mommy and the Orphanage

WHAT A DIFFICULT LIFE MY MOTHER HAD. FROM THE very beginning in 1914, adversity and challenges seemed to find her at every turn. Her indomitable spirit met each obstacle head on. Thank goodness she was blessed with extraordinary strength and a sense of loving kindness. She was the most courageous person I have ever known. She was my lifelong role model.

When she met the love of her life, my father, things looked up for a short while. Just as she was beginning to enjoy her good fortune, she was dealt yet another tragic hand.

Looking back, I consider my mother a miracle worker. How she managed to singlehandedly support our family of five on $3,000 a year in the late 1950s, I will never know. She was brilliant but never realized it. She always gave me credit for being the smart one, but it was she who was the genius. Following my father's stroke all those years ago, I became her copilot in navigating our family. Of course we were mother and daughter, but I also served as her confidante (those rare times that she would allow it) and co-caregiver for my father. On one hand, it was a simple mother/daughter relationship based on love, admiration, and respect. On the other, it was very complicated.

A beautiful woman with patrician bearing right up until the day she died at age ninety-four, my mother had a competitive edge when it came to appearance. Even though I looked a great deal like her, she would say things like, "It doesn't matter what you look like; what's important is that you are smart." From remarks like this, I intuited that I was not attractive and would need to rely on my intelligence to get ahead. This notion of unattractiveness was further confirmed when my adolescent self looked in the mirror and could only see acne, ugly blemishes that left me feeling embarrassed and humiliated. This skin condition, which started in my preteen years, lasted into my late twenties. And if the mirror wasn't enough to confirm the story, the lack of any attention from boys my age finished the job. Throughout high school, I was socially the gal pal: A generally well-liked and helpful person who did things like decorating for the junior and senior proms but never got to go. While that would all change much later, the pain of adolescence in those moments was real and left emotional scars for many years. But my scars couldn't begin to match what my mother endured.

Say the word *orphanage*, and you can see people get a look of great sadness, even pity. I hardly ever think about my years in the orphanage, but when I do, it's with good memories.

The people running my orphanage were kind and genteel. I was a serious and independent child, bordering on fresh, but the nuns and the ladies at the orphanage understood my barely three-year-old self and made me feel safe and welcome.

For nine years, Papa came to visit me every Saturday, and I would see the pain in his eyes each time he had to say goodbye. I know he wanted to pick me up and take me with him, but the state wouldn't let him. My three older brothers, initially placed in a different orphanage where child abuse was rampant, repeatedly begged to leave and were eventually allowed to go home. There they could earn money working odd jobs, including being golf caddies for the likes of Al Capone. An interesting education for boys all under the age of eleven.

I really don't remember my mother, Angelina, or my baby sister, Anita. Mama must have been an angel, just like her name, because while taking care of my ailing uncle (her younger brother), she and my sister both die of tuberculosis, or maybe it was the Spanish flu. I remember at about three years old walking behind a horse-drawn sleigh carrying their coffins.

When I am about five, I remember standing by the gate of the orphanage, where a nine-year-old boy is doing some yard work. He politely asks, "Do you know a girl named Mary DeStefano?"

My fresh answer is, "Who wants to know?"

He tells me that she is his sister, who would be about my age, and he hasn't seen her since she was very little and really wants to see her again. That's how I am reintroduced to my brother Charlie.

I am twelve when Papa comes for me. From this rather refined setting, I am brought to a cold-water flat, complete with heated bricks in winter to keep my feet warm. Not a happy day. I know my family is glad to finally have me back, but sometimes it is difficult for me not to wish to be back at the orphanage with its finery and order.

My three brothers, Ralph, Charlie, and Joe, whom I grow to adore, frighten me at first. The oldest, Ralph, who becomes a celebrated golf pro and is tragically incinerated in a car accident before he turns thirty, acts like I am his personal maid. Doing dishes, ironing, cleaning—that is not how I am used to spending my days. Sensitive brother Charlie idolizes Ralph and lives in his shadow. Then there is Joe, the brother closest to me in age, who is kind and generous and takes care of everyone.

Even Papa looks up to Joe. While as teenagers Ralph and Charlie leave our New Jersey home to become golf pros in Poughkeepsie, New York, Joe stays behind to take care of Papa. Papa is a hard-working man with Cary Grant good looks, and his escape from reality is to go to the local bars in Orange with his pals, much of the time counting on Joe to put him to bed when he returns. Then there are Papa's frequent card games in our flat, complete with cigarette butts, endless wine bottles from Papa's homemade bathtub batches, and the mess left behind for me to clean up.

Life at home is much harder than at the orphanage, and I often find myself daydreaming. Maybe I will soon meet my Prince Charming?

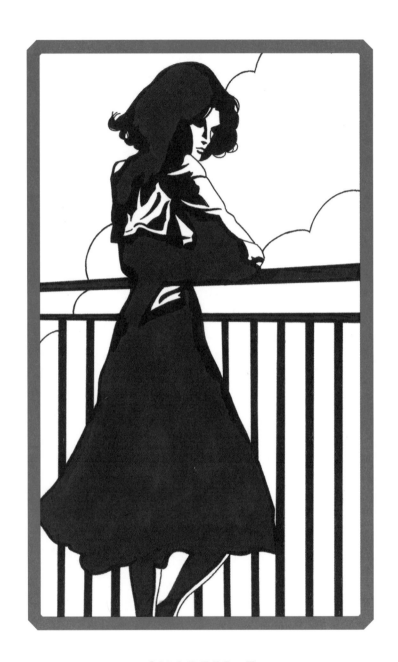

CHAPTER 7

Daddy Falls in Love

MY HANDSOME, WAVY-HAIRED FATHER WAS A TOTAL romantic who adored my mother. At the sight of her, his smile could light up an entire room. No matter what life would present, his palpable love for her would never change. As a first-generation Italian, his ties to family were strong and superseded everything. Important in his life were love, loyalty, and living honestly. Add respect, kindness, and a belief in God, and you have the principles by which he lived.

was seriously thinking about becoming a priest. That all changed the instant I saw her—she stood out as a fresh and natural beauty, and my heart began to speak.

We meet on a mystery bus ride in 1943. Mystery rides are popular and lots of adults in their twenties and thirties gather at the local YMCA in Orange, New Jersey, to be driven to an undisclosed location where, over cocktails, you get to meet new people. My brother and I have decided to try it.

Everything happens quickly. On the bus, I look over at her and smile, she smiles back. I introduce myself as Lou Falcone, we begin to chat, and I quickly realize how private and reserved she is. I keep trying to think of which movie actress she reminds me of, and then it comes to me—Rita Hayworth. She has the same beautiful smile and perfect teeth. Her eyes are wistful, bordering on slightly mischievous, and her tall silhouette is striking. And from the stylish way she's dressed, I gather she loves beautiful clothes.

She tells me that she lives nearby with her father, has two married brothers and that a third brother has recently died. When I ask about her mother, she says, "I have no memory of her; she died when I was very little."

I volunteer, "My brother and I live in Harrison over my parents' grocery store, and we have two older brothers who are already married. I'm a mechanical engineer, but I think I'm heading toward a job in sales. I love interacting with people." I purposely neglect to mention the priesthood.

While I can't figure out how old she is, my guess is mid-twenties just like me. She has been working for several years at an office job that she took right after high school, so my calculations are probably right.

I really want to see her again. At the end of the trip, as we are about to part ways, I ask if I can get in touch with her and perhaps invite her to dinner. She says that would be lovely.

On our first official date, she confesses it was my smile that attracted her.

Many dates and many months later, I'm sure she's the woman I want to marry, the perfect woman to be the mother of my children. I propose, and it's the happiest moment of my life when Mary DeStefano says, "Yes."

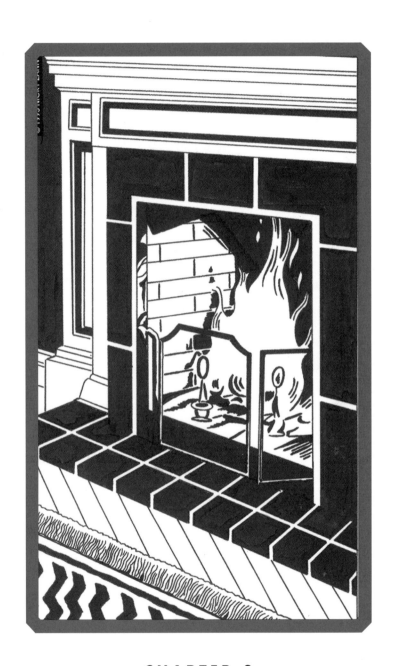

CHAPTER 8

Mommy's Dream
Comes True

ALL MY MOTHER EVER WANTED IN LIFE WAS TO BE married to a man she loved, who loved her right back. Add healthy children to the mix and perhaps a lovely home in the suburbs, and voilà, a perfect life. Her dream became reality . . . at least for a while.

I am so happy. My three children are wonderful—Mary Lou (ML), Louis, and Angel are all well behaved, smart, and talented to boot. My husband, Louie, is devoted to me and the children. Family means everything to him, as it does to me. People adore being around him. With his wit and charm, he's the life of every party.

Since I grew up without a mother, I want to make sure that I'm always there for my children, careful to give them everything I didn't have but also careful not to spoil them. Louie and I agree that good parenting means being both loving and strict.

It has never been easy for me to show emotion, so I don't hug and kiss a lot, even with my husband, who is always affectionate. I guess that's because displays of affection were frowned upon at the orphanage. But that's now behind me, and today my life is the one I dreamed about all those years ago.

If only this could last forever.

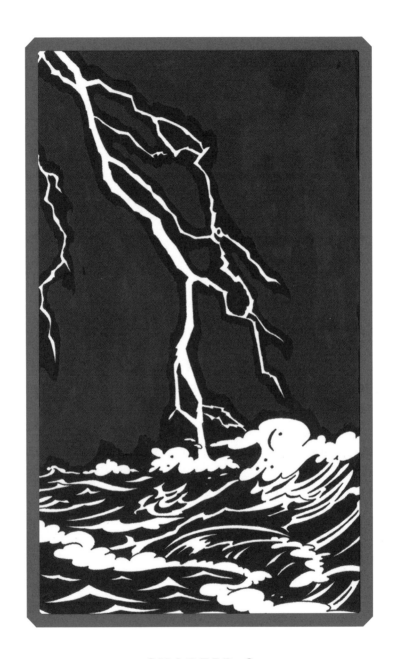

CHAPTER 9

Daddy's Nightmare

AS A DEVOUT CATHOLIC, MY FATHER HAD UNQUESTIONED faith in God. He was a man of infinite patience, and he had a will of iron when it came to protecting and providing for his wife and family. He was a strong person, both in character and physically, and he had never been sick a day in his life. His strength and stamina knew no boundaries. He worked hard, and he played hard. He was a gregarious man, universally loved and full of fun . . . and when appropriate, he could be deadly serious. Family and friends knew they could always count on Lou Falcone.

The dream couldn't last. It's 1955, and Mary and I have been married for eleven years.

Suddenly I'm trapped in a body that won't listen to my commands. I keep seeing the tunnel and the light, but I can't move. My children need me; I have to fight my way back from this debilitating stroke.

My brain is saying all the right things, or at least I think it is. I just cannot make the commands work.

Walk—I can't.

Move your right arm—I can't.

Speak—I can't. But I must.

Fight, fight, fight, never give up!

I fight to walk. It takes months, but I do it. At thirty-seven, I'm young and strong, I have to do this. It's slow. It's one step, literally, at a time. Months go by—I walk, albeit with a bad limp, but that doesn't matter. I'm mobile.

But I can't speak. I know what I want to say, but can't seem to form the words, much less sentences. Here the damage from the stroke turns out to be extensive and irreversible, but the attending physicians in Livingston, our small, northern New Jersey town, don't realize this and insist that we keep trying. After two years at the rehab center and just as the insurance money is running out, some well-meaning therapist tells my eleven-year-old daughter, ML, that because she is bright and capable, she should work with me daily on my speech.

I continue to be trapped in my silence, but now I must watch the anguish of my child, who wants so badly to help me. Here is my eldest being given an adult task. I am an adult who cannot make this work for her or for me. It breaks my heart to watch her earnestly trying and believing that she can do it.

I try and try—I fail. She tries and tries—she cannot make it happen. The truth, no one can. I hope she understands, it's not her fault.

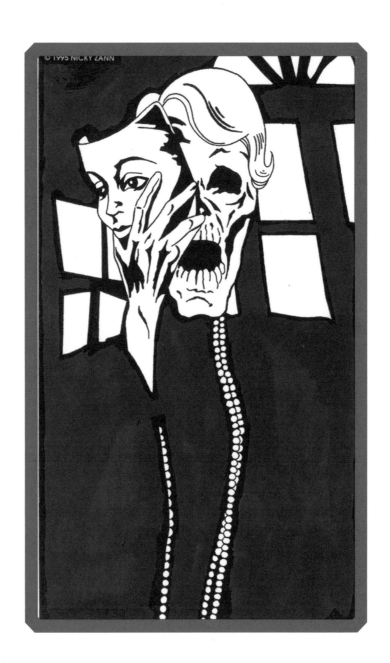

CHAPTER 10

Mommy's Heartbreak

HOW CLEARLY I REMEMBER THAT COLD DECEMBER DAY in 1955—sitting in the living room, enjoying the smell of baking cookies—when a loud crash from the kitchen startled me. Rushing toward the noise, I see freshly baked cookies scattered all over the floor, the metal cookie tray next to them, and glimpse my mother heading to the basement. Quietly creeping halfway down the cellar staircase, I watch and listen from a distance. I feel helpless, frozen in my tracks, just aching to put my arms around my beautiful mother and tell her, "Everything will be okay," as if I were the mother and she the child. My strong mother, the weight of the world on her shoulders, reduced to tears—so painful, a sight I had never before seen. I didn't approach her, I couldn't. She clearly needed to be alone, to finally express her pent-up feelings. Although almost seven decades have passed, I can still feel the heartbreak of that day.

I watch my wonderful husband struggling, young and in his prime, cut down by this massive stroke. Fate has just dealt an unexpected and cruel hand.

I have to be strong. I have to make everything work. The children must never worry. Only I know what's really happening—how long can I keep the stiff upper lip? Forever, I hope. I have to keep us together—family is everything.

Upon returning from the hospital, my Louie can't walk or talk. He is alive but in need of constant care. I am on my own.

My three children have their father—a blessing, though he must find new ways of communicating with all of us. Life is increasingly more difficult, and I have no one to turn to, no one to comfort me.

My eldest, ML, at age ten, is responsible beyond her years. Angel, my youngest, is an innocent five-year-old, and Louis, the middle child, a vulnerable seven.

After the initial sympathy and concern, relatives don't want to be burdened. Besides, I am a private person, especially about my feelings. In addition to being a wife, now caregiver, and a mother, I'm working three jobs: factory by day, bakery on weekends, babysitting several nights a week. I am about to explode. Christmas is coming, and it's important to have some sense of normalcy for the children.

As I prepare to bake cookies, the walls are closing in. My hands are shaking. I am nervous about so many things.

The cookie tray slips out of my hands onto the floor, and cookies scatter everywhere. I mustn't lose it in front of the children. For the first time in six months, I can't hold it in any longer.

Feeling desperately alone, I run to the basement, and I cry.

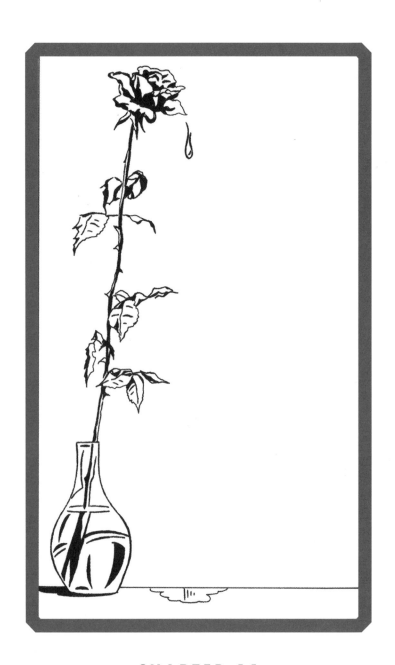

CHAPTER 11

I Grow Up Overnight

Everything around me is changing so fast. The year is 1955 and, at age ten, I'm suddenly blindsided by two new companions: fear and anger. Until now, my biggest problem was being called "fatso" on the playground.

I'm a Mommy's girl. I worship my mother and don't make a move without asking her first . . . even something silly like, "Mommy, if I'm too hot on the playground, should I take off my coat?"

A needy kid? Absolutely.

Then, almost overnight, I'm forced to change because I have to help take care of Daddy. No one tells me what to do or what to expect. I pray a lot for answers but have to make my own decisions. It's hard, and I feel alone. I understand it's my job to keep my brother and sister safe—I am grateful that at least they can confide in each other.

Everyone has new responsibilities. Mommy is working three jobs. We all have chores. The one I hate the most is having to ignite the gas oven pilot light with a match. I hate lighting matches, and the explosive sound of the pilot light catching fire always frightens me. I'm scared to death that I will blow up the house.

I listen extra hard to everything that's being said around me, but the adults are not sharing much information.

Then, the people at Daddy's rehab center ask me to do an important job, an adult's job. Daddy walked—now he must speak. They tell me I can help him and show me what to do. They give me workbooks to use. They give me flashcards with simple words, and some have complete sentences. Teaching Daddy doesn't feel right to me. I don't like it but I have no choice, I have to help. Can I do it? I really don't know.

While I understand how important it is to help Daddy, I admit I'm scared. Scared that I will fail, and I don't want to fail, especially not at this.

Daddy is uncomfortable. I am too. I work with him every day after school. I try and try to make him speak. He tries and tries— nothing. It's agony for him. The more I push him, the more I feel like a bully.

I see his frustration and, worse, I see his tears. My heart breaks. I have made my father cry, and I am not proud of that. The situation is hopeless; he will never speak. But no one has said that to either of us.

Sometimes I feel just plain lonely. Other times I feel sorry for myself, because I can't afford to do what my friends are doing— no time and no money. Where to turn? Grandpa, of course, but soon he too will be taken away from me to live with my Uncle Joe.

I want badly to go to Mommy and have her reassure me that everything will be okay. She is so busy. I just can't add to her troubles. I have to figure this out for myself.

One day, trying to be helpful, my Uncle Joe, my mother's favorite brother, takes my cousin Ruthie and me to the local Woolworth's, giving us each twenty-five cents to spend. I look at everything. There's nothing I want. Why? I suddenly understand that every penny counts. I keep looking at the twenty-five cents, holding onto its possibilities. If I don't spend it, I can save it; or someone else might need it. This is no time to be frivolous. So much seems to be invested in the twenty-five cents. I return home clutching the quarter, paralyzed by my inability to spend it. I save it.

A year later, watching how hard Mommy must work and how she is struggling to support our family, I find myself standing in front of the bathroom mirror vowing out loud, "I will never be poor." I am eleven years old.

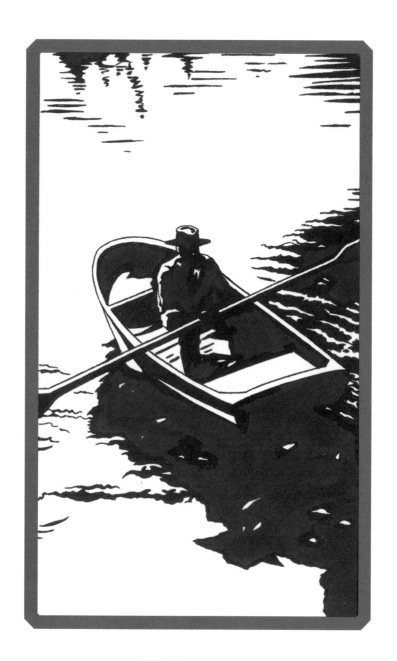

CHAPTER 12

Louis, My Brother

MY BROTHER, LOUIS, WAS A VERY SENSITIVE CHILD, and the one most severely affected by my father's illness. Just when a boy needs his dad's guidance the most, Louis couldn't turn to or count on him, nor did he have a significant male role model—no one stepped up to fill that void. Louis never quite knew where he fit in. It must have been equally painful for my father to watch and not be able to act. While my brother, as I've mentioned before, was my mother's favorite child, she was also very hard on him, insisting that he play sports like the other boys. But he had little to no interest in sports. What he loved was making everything look beautiful. He naturally gravitated to artistic pursuits like playing the violin and designing dresses for my sister's Barbie dolls. Unfortunately, these activities were often discouraged by my mother, but his artistic side prevailed. He became a top-notch graphic designer, running a successful business for many decades on the West Coast, where he felt free to be himself.

Early on I saw Louis's complete vulnerability, a vulnerability I shared but kept hidden. His youthful attempts at a conventional suburban way of life gave way to exploring a more relevant lifestyle. As a student at the Kansas City

Art Institute and thriving there, Louis found his way as an artist and became enlightened about his sexual orientation as well. It was not until the early-1970s, when he was in his early twenties, that he shared with my parents that he was gay. My mother, visibly taken by surprise, had an immediate and spontaneous reaction. Not missing a beat, she said: "I love you, you're my son. Your choice doesn't matter as long as it makes you happy. We won't love you any less." Privately she asked me if this was a phase that he might outgrow, but deep down she knew this was the natural path for Louis and accepted it. I saw from my father's loving expression, so did he. Several years later, in 1980, when my father was too ill to travel, my mother went to Louis's wedding in Los Angeles, years before gay marriage was accepted—and she had a great time! So did I as the maid of honor.

My only sadness is that Louis seems to have inherited my father's genes when it comes to being susceptible to illness, but he has also inherited his bravery.

I am seven years old, and because I don't understand what's happening, I'm always scared.

We kneel on my little sister Angel's bed, looking out of the second-story bedroom window, asking no one in particular, "Where are they taking our daddy in the white truck with the siren?" The three of us just hold hands, quietly watching, not even crying—just frightened.

I don't remember going to sleep that June night in 1955, but I must have. The next day we're told that Daddy is very sick, and Mommy is very busy, and we shouldn't bother her.

My older sister, ML, the soon-to-be-ten-year-old boss, is in charge. My little sister, Angel, who is just about to turn five and will not have a very happy birthday, doesn't understand anything that's going on, so she just hugs her toy monkeys.

Daddy's mother is always around and tries to help, but she wants to take over, and Mommy says, "No! I can do it myself."

Not even the doctor in our town has seen a stroke in someone Daddy's age. They treat him at home for three days for something they call dehydration. I hear someone say, "We don't think he's going to make it . . ."—that's when the white truck comes and takes him away.

Two months go by, and the white truck returns. This time it brings Daddy back, but he isn't the same. He can't walk, he can't talk. He smiles at us as they carry him into the house.

I recognize the smile. What I don't recognize are the ugly sounds he's making. What scares me the most is when he starts to shake and white stuff comes out of his mouth. I run from the house and hide in the front bushes until I think it's safe to come out.

I feel guilty that I'm hiding, guilty that I want my real father back and not this stranger, guilty that I feel helpless. I'm so scared. I'm angry at Daddy for leaving me to be the man of the house.

I love Daddy, and then sometimes I hate him. He has let me down. I am a skinny little kid, bullied and beaten up by the older, mean kids as I walk home alone from school. It doesn't help that I'm carrying a violin case. The bullies are only too happy to throw the case into the snow first and then me after it. Not fitting in anywhere and having no one to really turn to except my sisters, I try running away a few times, but of course, I always come back—where would I go?

I know that none of this is my fault, but why do I still feel guilty?

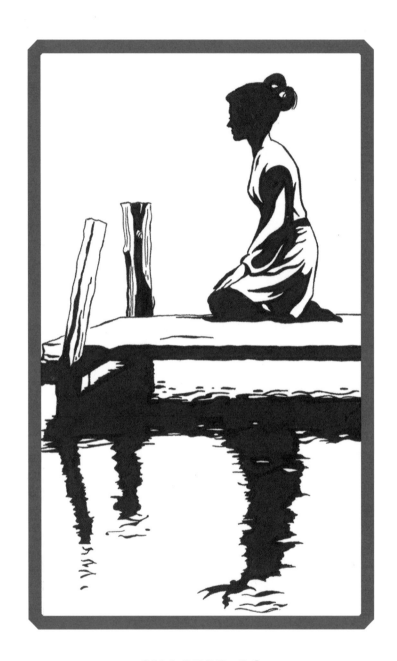

CHAPTER 13

Angel,
My Little Sister

AS A CHILD, MY SISTER ANGELA, KNOWN TO ALL AS Angel, took on the role of my father's protector and remained steadfast in that role until he died in 1981 from cancer—multiple myeloma, to be exact. He was sixty-four years old, and since age thirty-seven had been unable to speak. He managed to find alternate ways to communicate, some successful and some not. He would point or slowly write a word or underline something in the newspaper . . . but what was he thinking? Between him and my mother, there definitely was telepathy and infinite patience; and we children got pretty good at intuiting, but we were kids, and patience was not always our strong suit. We never heard a complete sentence from him, much less a paragraph, so what he thought or how he felt had to be surmised from his body language and from his kind and loving eyes, which told most of the story. How horrible it must have been for him to be utterly trapped. And yet, if he was frustrated, and surely he must have been, he hardly ever let us see it. I think he was grateful to be alive, grateful for his family, and grateful that we stuck together, protecting one another and him. That omnipresent smile that he had for everyone and almost every situation was real, and despite everything he had to endure, he possessed the most positive spirit I have ever encountered.

My father's greatest joy in his last years was his only grandchild, my sister's daughter, Stephanie. Angel made sure my father was included in protecting and nurturing Stephanie, and a beautiful bond was forged. He adored Steph, and she loved her "Poppy." Whenever she was with him, no matter how much pain he was in from the cancer, his big smile and warm hugs were there for her. The newest addition to our family was the apple of Poppy's eye, and being with his beautiful granddaughter made his last days happy ones.

Angel's life has been that of a gifted mother and great supporter of others, with our parents at the top of the list. As a popular teenager about to graduate high school, she gave up her scholarship to college, a combination of not wanting to burden our parents who couldn't afford to help and having a serious boyfriend. Her high school sweetheart won out, and they married. Before divorcing him, she endured sixteen difficult years as the wife of a raging alcoholic. Protecting her daughter above all, she supported her family for decades as a paralegal. Following in our mother's footsteps, Angel had a talent for sewing and other needlework, which she turned into a cottage industry. Angel's support of her daughter, Stephanie DePalma, has never waned.

Today Stephanie is a filmmaker, specializing in documentary films. In fact, her very first documentary film was *Ralph: Someone to Me*, a film profiling her late father and his disease of alcoholism. As a fitting tribute to Steph's talent and her capacity for love and forgiveness, the film won Best Directorial Debut at the New York International Film

Festival in 2010. We were all there to cheer her on, with
Poppy applauding from heaven.

Yes, Angel's my name, and, yes, I love it—what kid wouldn't
with everyone constantly calling out *Angel.* Makes me feel
very special. How lucky for me that Mommy wanted to honor
her mother.

What do I remember from my earliest days? Not too much:
being cuddled by Mommy, adored by Daddy (I was always his
favorite), accepted by my brother and his friends as the tagalong,
and looked after by my big sister.

As I turn five, with everything swirling around me, I can only
talk to Big Jock, Middle Jock, and my closest friend, Little Jock,
the puppet. My toy monkeys are always there for me.

My sister, ML, and I pray a lot, especially at church. This is
important to Daddy. My brother, Louis, and Mommy don't care
much about church. Mommy says you can pray anywhere.

I never give anyone any trouble and do what I am told. While
I don't understand what is going on, I do feel loved and protected. I watch and I notice things, things that really bother me,
like conversations at the dinner table where everyone talks only
to Mommy. I know that Daddy can't talk, but he's never included
and often forgotten. This makes me feel bad for him, so I decide
that I am going to be Daddy's protector, a role I silently promise
to play forever.

I guess everybody in my family feels like a protector of some
kind. My big sister and my brother protect me, while our mother
works all the time to protect the whole family.

Our sister loves us but is very bossy. One day, during a terrible
snow and ice storm, my sister can't find us. She's very worried and
traces the path back to our school. Not finding us, she starts the
return to our house, and on the very steep hill, she falls and hits

the ice, jaw first. The tables are now turned, and we find her—her mouth frozen shut so she can't boss us around. At first, we think this is funny, and then we stop laughing when we realize she's really hurt. Taking her to our neighbor's house for help, we feel guilty and frightened. We know from the look in her eyes that she too is frightened, and this is something she has never let us see before. She's always in charge, hiding what she really feels, just like Mommy. A few hours later, her jaw thaws out and she can talk. What a relief to have our bossy sister back.

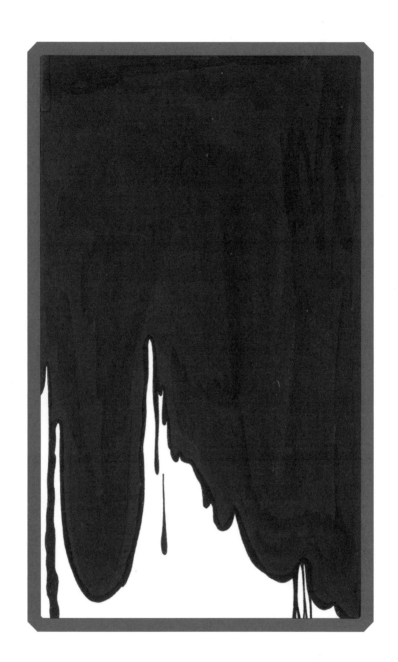

CHAPTER 14

Farewell to Daddy

Fear is an ever-present factor when, as a child, you sense that a situation beyond your control could become complicated and dangerous. Unbeknownst to my brother, Louis, my sister, Angel, and me, we as children shared a common fear: that our father would encounter a situation in which he might come to harm because he was unable to speak. Mercifully he was never harmed, but that fear lingered for all of us until after his death.

Throughout childhood, we three siblings often felt conflicted. Mostly we felt compassion for our father; sometimes we felt pity, and occasionally we felt embarrassed.

For more than twenty-five years, Daddy was held hostage by the aftermath of his massive stroke. What a fighter he was. Thanks to his unshakable spirit, he learned to walk again, but not to speak. The brain damage from the stroke was extensive, especially in the area of the brain that controls speech. No one seems to have realized how extensive it was. From age thirty-seven on, he never had the chance verbally to share his thoughts and feelings with anyone—not Mommy, not the three of us. Daddy, once the life of the party, became the smiling, aware, but silent observer.

He would utter isolated words here and there. One day at dinner, we were talking about dogs in the neighborhood, and Angel asked about a specific animal. Out of nowhere Daddy said, "mongrel," certainly not your everyday word.

What we remember most is his never-ending smile. But we also remember some terrifying moments, like the time Daddy took Louis to the Department of Motor Vehicles to get his learner's permit.

As Louis tells it: "I am sixteen and so excited to be getting my driver's permit. As Daddy gets out of the car, the inspectors notice that he is walking with a considerable limp. Two very mean-spirited officers immediately isolate Daddy in a room and refuse to let me in. I am frantic, on the verge of a panic attack trying to tell them that my father can't talk, and I have to be with him. It's a horrible moment, and I can't begin to imagine how Daddy is feeling, utterly helpless to defend himself. While in hindsight I know he probably should not have been driving, in that moment the inspectors are clearly very aware. Between Daddy's right arm, which does not work, and his right foot, which drags, we all are sensing a disaster waiting to happen. After begging the DMV inspectors to let me be with him, they finally let me in. Revoking Daddy's license on the spot, they say, 'If you get a left foot gas pedal installed, bring the car back here for inspection, and pass a new driving test, we will give your license back.' While this incident traumatized me, I will never know what it did to Daddy. But being determined, Daddy miraculously got his driver's license back, and yes, I got my driver's permit too."

Daddy loved life, even though it robbed him just as he was about to hit his prime. You'd think that after years of adversity, nothing more could be taken from him. Well, the universe had more in store. One day, he rolled over in bed and broke his arm, just by rolling over. What is going on? He is hospitalized and the doctors test and test. For almost two years, his low-grade fever will not break, and the spinal taps are painful and endless.

The final diagnosis is multiple myeloma, a cancer of the blood that builds up in the bone marrow. When Daddy hears the diagnosis, his face drops. The famous smile vanishes, and he, who is such a devout believer in God, utters, "God—*pfff.*" This is the final straw: He has lost hope. After all that he has endured, to have this death sentence added to his living hell is just too much, even for this steadfast believer.

We three, with our mother's blessing, finally tell the doctors: "Enough is enough. Stop using him as a human pin cushion. Please give him some peace and dignity."

With the prodding and poking stopped, he seems relieved as he drifts in and out of consciousness. At one point toward the end of July 1981, with all of us gathered in his hospital room, I say: "We are all here, Daddy. We love you, and you deserve to rest. If you want to let go, it's okay. We promise to look out for one another and to protect Mommy."

Angel, her heart breaking, nods in agreement. Louis, who just can't resist a moment of truth coupled with a bit of levity, pipes up and says, "You see, Daddy, Mary Lou has always been bossy, and she's still telling us what to do."

Thanks to Louis's quip, Daddy opens his eyes and we get to see his famous smile one last time . . . and then, he is gone.

Years later, in speaking about our fears, we three realize that until the day our father died at age sixty-four, we lived in fear of something like the DMV incident or worse happening. When he died, we shared a sense of relief that he was finally at peace and no longer vulnerable. Our fear for him, present since childhood, was lifted. It was replaced by a profound sadness: Angel's sadness that ultimately she had not been able to protect Daddy and that he would never see his baby granddaughter grow up; Louis's sadness that he never had the father/son relationship that he craved; and my sadness that I had not been able to help Daddy communicate his thoughts and feelings through words.

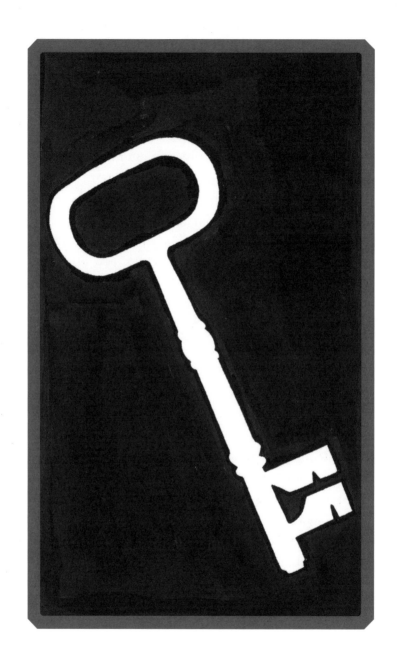

CHAPTER 15

My Passport to the World

MUSIC BECAME MY PASSPORT TO THE WORLD.

Around the time of my father's stroke, when I was about ten, I noticed that when I sang "Bless This House," all the adults in the room would be wiping away tears. What a revelation—this was power, the power of music to move people while freeing myself to unselfconsciously share my emotions. It was okay to be emotional when speaking through music, where in everyday life I wouldn't dare. I recognized this as a gift and took the responsibility of this gift very seriously, grateful to have it.

Soon, voices of importance and authority were listening and becoming my champions—the superheroes to whom I pay tribute in this chapter. The first was Roy Lenox, my high school music teacher who opened windows and doors I never knew existed. In fast succession followed my first voice teacher, Dorothy Fulmer, and a bit later Efrem Zimbalist Sr., director of the Curtis Institute of Music.

THE HIGH SCHOOL MUSIC TEACHER

High school for some is the ultimate experience, while for others it can be just plain painful. For me it was a wonderful time of academic growth and a time of discovery that became the cornerstone for my future. Not belonging to any high school clique, I was admired by some, tolerated by others, and downright disliked by those who were jealous.

We often hear about that special educator who makes a difference, and I was lucky enough to encounter that person. Leroy "Roy" Lenox was a father figure and, yes, I had a teenage crush on him. He was the first person with whom I could have deep conversations about life. He enriched my world, encouraging me to aim high.

He and I remained close throughout my high school years and stayed friends throughout his life. I knew his family and became friendly with his youngest daughter whom he adored. Fifty years after high school, during a visit with his daughter, she confided in me: "You probably sensed that my father was pretty unhappy at home, and I wanted so much to see him happy. Even as a kid, I knew that when you were around, he was definitely happy. It was clear to me, he loved you." Then she added, "May I ask you a personal question? Did you and my father ever have an affair?"

My answer, "A physical affair, no. An affair of the heart, yes."

As we start the glee club rehearsal, I am startled by a voice soaring above the others. Who is it? I look around and see that the voice belongs to a tall newcomer, someone who clearly loves to sing.

I speak with her after class and decide to break one of my own rules. I invite this freshman to audition for the select vocal ensemble open only to upper classmen. Of course I admit her to the group.

She blushes a lot and I find her to be rather shy, but along with the shyness comes a quiet confidence—an interesting combination. She intrigues me.

I look forward to seeing her in the hallways, in the classroom, at practice sessions after school. Occasionally, I offer her a ride home.

The occasional ride becomes the norm. We talk about everything. She is smart and pragmatic and, I discover, much older than her years. Often I forget that I am talking to a teenager and not a peer.

We talk about her life, her path. She tells me that she wants to be a math teacher, but slowly I begin to introduce thoughts about possibly teaching music or even becoming a performer.

Her aunt and uncle seek me out and ask: "How far can our niece go? Is she really that talented?" Normally these would be questions posed by parents, but I know that her father is incapacitated, and her mother is so busy holding down multiple jobs that she doesn't have time for anything else. No one at school has any idea what this family is dealing with.

My instinct is to share all that I can with this teenager and to protect her from potential show business nonsense. I tell her real-life horror stories from friends currently performing on Broadway, stories about bad people posing as do-gooders in order to ultimately sabotage and destroy talent. "Jealousy knows no boundaries," I tell her.

I give her every opportunity to shine, while being careful not to overdo it.

Gradually she's becoming my muse. I talk about her constantly to my family, to my friends. I have her sing for everyone I know. She brings us all joy.

Our rides home continue and last for hours as we sit in my car talking and talking. I sense that she enjoys these moments as much as I do.

Her mother often asks what on earth a young girl and a fifty-year-old man could possibly talk about for that many hours. Her answer, "Life!"

And life it is. She makes me feel more alive than I have in years.

I encourage her to choose a life in music. Knowing that she has no financial resources, I suggest that, along with applying to local colleges (which would accept her in an instant), she might audition for a special music school in Philadelphia, the Curtis Institute of Music. This all-scholarship school accepts very few, and while it's a long shot, I think she's got what it takes. Even though famous musicians like Leonard Bernstein have gone there, she has never heard of the school.

She may be shy, but she does love a challenge. Yes, she will try.

FIRST VOICE TEACHER

> In my early teens, I longed for some escape from reality, and working with my first voice teacher, Dorothy Fulmer, was a welcome release from my worries. For a few hours each week, I could just get lost in the music. She was an inspiration, never giving up on her fight for life, even when her body, crippled by multiple sclerosis, completely betrayed her, and all she could do was blink one eye. Her courage was equal to my father's. They were both dealt impossible cards and inspired me with their determination.

The doorbell rings. My wheelchair is stuck, preventing me from opening the door. A cheery soprano "Hello, come in" will have to do.

In walks a tall, slim girl with excellent posture and a warm smile that makes me look past her severe acne. She sings "Bless This House" and the Schubert "Ave Maria." I fight back tears as I wonder how this fifteen-year-old could possibly infuse this music with so much emotion and pathos.

Her voice is beautiful and very mature—she sounds more like a thirty-year-old who has lived a full life. Even though she has a natural reserve, she is not afraid to reveal herself through the music.

Once, I aspired to be a professional singer. Now, thanks to multiple sclerosis, I am cemented to the chair that serves as my legs. I pin my hopes on her and want her to succeed in the profession I longed to pursue.

After she's no longer my student, she doesn't forget me. She takes me on her journey, calling frequently to give me updates and regaling me with stories. Even when I am completely bedridden, unable to even whisper her name, she visits.

Clearly her singing voice is her God-given gift, but as I tell her, her gifts of communication and compassion are equally important.

DIRECTOR, THE CURTIS INSTITUTE OF MUSIC

I will never know: Did I somehow remind Efrem Zimbalist Sr., director of the Curtis Institute, of his first wife, the famous opera singer Alma Gluck? This is quite a bold and presumptuous thought on my part, but I have always wondered. What I do know is that his intervention at my Curtis audition changed the course of my life, and I will be forever grateful.

In my student days, surrounded at Curtis by the best, I had an epiphany. I too needed to be the best; but even then, I was pretty sure it wasn't going to be as a singer. Don't get me wrong, I loved music and I loved performing, but in my heart, I knew I would never be the best in this arena. Why? Quite simply because I didn't need to

sing more than anything in the world. And to succeed as
a singer or as a performer of any kind, you must need it
above everything—and I do mean everything. Wanting it
is never enough. What was crystal clear to me was that
I needed to communicate. What form that would take
remained to be seen. And so, the search for my true calling
began, even while still a student at Curtis.

The violin is so like the human voice, and I love both instruments.
My late wife was a glorious singer, an international star. Often
when we played duets in concerts, voice and violin as one, I
would feel totally content and complete. She was taken from me
too early. I remarried a wonderful, generous woman, but my first
wife remains the love of my life.

As director of Philadelphia's Curtis Institute of Music, I occasionally sit in on auditions other than violin. This year, it's voice
auditions that interest me.

Even though the East Coast has just been hit by a late April
blizzard, the 1963 auditions go on as planned. It is mid-morning
on day two of auditions, and we have heard a few nice voices. Our
fifth candidate is only seventeen. Normally we do not allow students that young to audition in voice, but her high school music
teacher has written such a compelling letter, we are curious to
hear her.

Tall and regal, she enters the grand room. She starts with an
obscure song by Galuppi, and then we choose the Rachmaninoff
song, "O Thou Billowy Harvest Field."

At the piano is my longtime friend and colleague Vladimir
Sokoloff, a brilliant musician. She hands him a handwritten man-
uscript (yes, she has hand-copied every note of the Galuppi song),
which has a full-page introduction. To save time, he starts the
introduction a few measures before the vocal line begins.

At the conclusion of this now shortened introduction, she calmly turns to him saying, "Excuse me, sir, but I need to hear the entire introduction to properly get into the song." Quietly chuckling to himself, he suspects no one in her small town has been able to play the intricate introduction. She probably just wants the opportunity to hear it played through by a professional, so, he obliges.

This gets my attention, and I now watch and listen carefully. What she shares is truly beautiful. Her serenity and sincerity draw you in, compel you to listen. When she moves on to the Rachmaninoff song, I am deeply touched. These are my roots she is singing about, my homeland. My thoughts go to many happy times, happy places, and to my first wife, Alma Gluck.

Graciously thanking us for the opportunity, she leaves. We hear singers for the next several days, but her audition stays with me. Out of hundreds, we can choose only two. We are a very small school, with 150 students total, mostly instrumentalists and only twenty singers.

Never before have I interfered with the voice teachers' choices. This time is different. I tell them that I want this seventeen-year-old in the school, and I will personally choose her teacher. Sokoloff and I have worked together for decades. We agree that this young girl will be one of the greats, even though we are the only ones at the audition who share this opinion.

September comes and she has no idea why or how she was chosen. I encounter her occasionally on the grand staircase that leads to my studio. She respectfully smiles and nods, as do I. We never speak. I make sure to attend her recitals, silently monitoring her progress. She matures nicely, and after three years, at age twenty, she graduates and starts her singing career.

Years later, I give her voice teacher, Eufemia Giannini Gregory, permission to tell her about how she was chosen to be part of the Curtis legacy.

LOUIS, ANGEL, AND THE ENVELOPE, PLEASE

> As a trio, my brother, my sister, and I to this day delight in one another's triumphs. We have stayed close in good times and in times of stress, sadness, illness, and hardship, blessed to have one another. "Family is everything," our mother would say, and we would all chuckle at the phrase, rolling our eyes with a "there she goes again" smirk. Well, guess what? She was right.

Our big sister, ML, leaves for the church with our parents at around 10:00 a.m. She is always in demand for singing at weddings, a specialty of hers. Today is one of those days.

When the mail arrives, we look at each other: Should we or shouldn't we? In the pile is a letter from Curtis, where she has just auditioned.

Going to Philadelphia last week was the biggest trip of her life. She came home that same day, raving about this man who played the piano for her. She told us how he had inspired her to sing better than she knew how. "No matter what happens," she said, "I have had the thrill of a lifetime. What an extraordinary experience!"

Now, on this beautiful Saturday morning, we are holding her life in our hands—do we dare? We really want to know. Well, we could use the tea kettle to steam open the letter, read what it has to say, and re-glue the envelope. We have about an hour before she comes home. If we are careful, she will never know. Angel finally says, "Oh, come on, let's live dangerously and go for It."

We are the first to know. Her dream has come true. We jump up and down, so excited for our big sister. Now, back to acting normal.

When she returns from church, we are casually sitting in the kitchen, eyes glued to the mail now placed on the dining room table. We were careful to put her letter on the top of the pile so she can't miss it. We wait, trying to keep our excitement contained. Will she suspect what we've done?

The look of disbelief as she reads her acceptance letter makes us want to cry. She never expected to be chosen and, for once, with tears of joy streaming down her face, ML is speechless.

I'M ON THE ROAD TO CURTIS AND BEYOND

During my teenage years and before I got to Curtis, there were many lessons to be learned from working a variety of jobs—the greatest lesson being the difference between a job and a career.

My worst job, bar none, actually turned out to be a major lesson in disguise. Most people have never heard of an interception operator. Well, Ma Bell, which once had a national telephone monopoly, used to have such a job. In the 1960s, this was the person who told you that the number you were calling had been disconnected. In other words, the person whose voice no one ever wants to hear. That person for two very long summers was me. During what felt like an eight-hour-a-day prison sentence, customers yelled and screamed obscenities, and when I objected saying, "Excuse me, sir/madam, language of this kind is never allowed in my home," a member of the head operator's "Gestapo" team would reprimand me for being rude, thus giving new meaning to the phrase, "The customer is always right." Why did I stay in such an abusive job? It paid the handsome sum of $47 per week, and I needed the money for school. Even though I was going to an all-scholarship school—the Curtis Institute—food and rent (no dorms) in Philadelphia needed to be paid by me.

The dreadful telephone company experience gave me an early insight into the importance of finding a career versus a job. I became determined to identify a career that would excite me every morning. A tall order, yes, and it would take me ten years to find it.

Even as a kid, I thought about being entrepreneurial. My first business at age eleven was babysitting. This didn't take too much imagination as I already had lots of practice in my own family—so much so, that down the road, I knew I didn't need to have my own children.

The next stop was waitressing at the local diner. But given my natural clumsiness, this position proved disastrous, and I was promptly promoted to hostess—a much better fit. The best job ever during my high school days was singing at weddings and funerals, allowing me to pay for my voice lessons; plus I discovered it's pure heaven to be paid for something you love to do.

Many crazy and varied jobs followed over the years, all sharing a common theme: learning on the job.

Daydreaming, a frequent activity for me, evolved into the art of visualizing, a major tool that I still use today. If I can imagine or see it, then feel it, and then act on it, I can do it. This, coupled with fierce determination, self-motivation, and hard work, has been a winning combination. I often jokingly state that self-employment was my only option, because who in the world would want me in their midst full-time?

Have I been a risk taker over the years? Yes, but the risks have been carefully visualized, researched, and planned. Truth be told, there are times when I have relied on pure instinct and a large leap of faith, my heart pounding the whole time.

I feel very blessed that the wings of fate have carried me through many training-on-the-job adventures that eventually morphed into fulfilling careers.

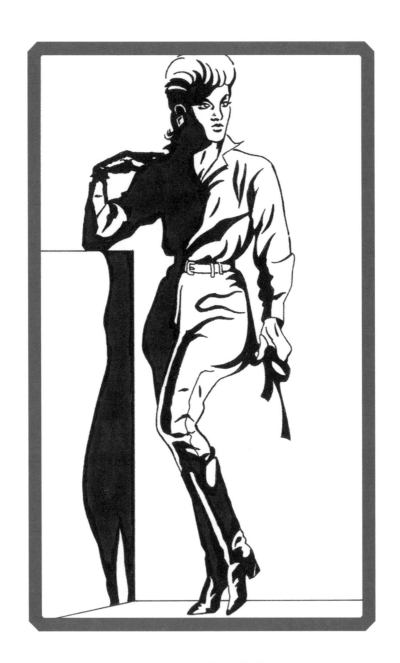

CHAPTER 16

First Love, an Important Audition, and the Dissolution of Both

The Curtis Institute experience begins. My first days in Philadelphia are miserable and lonely, filled with reticence and intimidation. With no dorms or school community center, I feel completely isolated, living in an apartment I can barely afford. Do I really belong here? More often than not, I find myself in tears, praying in a nearby church, asking for an answer to this question.

Being at Curtis feels like being on a movie set. Here is this beautiful, old, Center City Philadelphia mansion on Rittenhouse Square, where strains of glorious music pour out from the studios of famous faculty members and from the practice rooms of fellow students, all adding to my lack of confidence, which I do my very best to hide. Among the friendlier and more welcoming class-mates is a popular, good-looking, young organist, John Binsfeld, who is in the class one year ahead of me. Thank goodness for a kind smile and warm hello every now and then. After a few weeks, which felt like an eternity, the spell of intimidation and loneliness suddenly lifts.

Little did I realize in those early days just how major a role John Binsfeld would be playing in my life.

It started on a blustery March day in 1964. The young members of the Cherub Choir are captivated, all vying for the Pied Piper's attention. These adoring five- and six-year-olds are singing their little hearts out, eager to please the tall, effervescent man who leads them. My classmate John Binsfeld has hired me to sing for the Sunday service in this rural Pennsylvania church. I'm early for my rehearsal, so, I watch. Until this moment, I haven't given this classmate much thought.

Out of nowhere, I feel like I've been hit by a thunderbolt. A wave of intense emotion fills me. I feel passion, love, first love! It surprises me, and I rush home to my roommates, declaring that I am in love. Because I am younger than my roommates by several years, they find my revelation amusing, but also a bit annoying.

This takes place during the second half of my freshman year at Curtis. By the beginning of my second year, John is my first real boyfriend, my beau. We share thoughts and dreams and fears with one another in a stream of never-ending conversation. Not since the days with my high school music teacher, Roy Lenox, have I felt so connected to another person.

John is magical and charismatic. Everyone loves him. I love him! He's a great talent and has recently started a new church position as organist and choirmaster at Christ Church, the most historic church in the City of Brotherly Love. He hires me as his soprano soloist, and making music with him is a highlight of every week. We are inseparable; emotionally and spiritually, we speak the same language. All this perfection, yet we never consummate the relationship. My passion is soaring, but no matter what I do or say, he won't allow anything beyond kissing and hugging.

It's Christmas 1964, and John presents me with an exquisite double-strand pearl necklace from Nan Duskin, the most exclusive store in Philadelphia. I am totally surprised and, of course, utterly delighted. Following the Christmas Eve service at Christ Church, I go back to my Philadelphia apartment alone. Everyone else has scattered. I won't be going home to New Jersey until Christmas Day.

As I put on my blue lace negligee, feeling beautiful and dreamy, I look at myself in the bathroom mirror, the exquisite pearls gracing my throat. If only he could see me like this, but . . . the recognition that flashes through my mind shocks me: John is gay.

John's gift of pearls turns out to be symbolic in more ways than just that Christmas Eve revelation.

The following year, during an audition in New York City before the Fulbright Scholarship Committee, I am feeling well put together in my lovely, simple, A-line, hot pink audition dress, adorned with my stunning "good luck" pearls. I am halfway through the first aria when I stop the show, and not with my singing! The pearls have broken and are scattering all over the stage around my feet, rolling off the platform, aiming directly for the judges' table. Oh, my God—what now? When the judges stop laughing, the chairman of the jury, Martial Singher, whom I happen to know from Curtis, says in his very thick French accent, "Well, my dear, too bad you are not singing 'The Jewel Song.'"

Needless to say, the audition is a disaster, and no, I didn't get the Fulbright.

Those pearls turn out to be a metaphor for my life at that moment: fragile with portentous overtones. My very special "first love" is coming to an end, romantically breaking apart, but John Binsfeld and I continue to love one another for life.

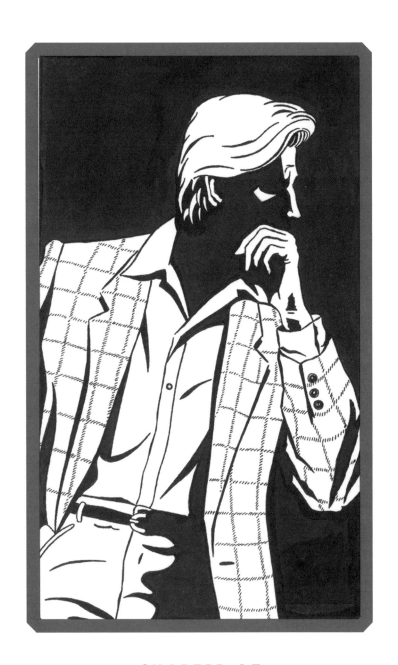

CHAPTER 17

Forever Connected

What is it about ML? I can't put my finger on it. Recently, I hired her to come to my hometown church for Palm Sunday to sing "I know that my Redeemer liveth" from the *Messiah*. Everyone was speechless. Great voice, yes, but the conviction with which she sings makes you a believer too. Since that spring day in 1964, I have not been able to listen to anyone else sing this without hearing her.

There is something special about this girl, yet I am fighting all sorts of feelings. I can't stop thinking about her. While I am drawn to her light, my dark side keeps pulling at me. Still, I want ML in my life; I want her.

I embrace her, I take her in my arms, I passionately kiss her, and I stop.

Flings, there have been many, and there will be others. As much as I love her, I will not whisk her off to bed or offer her any hope for a future. I know she is hungry for this, but I cannot. ML is too precious to me; this love is pure and must stay that way.

For the better part of two years, she is a major part of my life—I cannot live without her, and I cannot bring myself to live with her.

Personal and professional conflict rages within me. Had I not been conflicted, I might have become a priest. My calling is becoming clearer. A ministry, yes, but through music. Having recently been appointed minister of music at the most historic and prestigious church in Philadelphia, I know I can make a difference. With this ministry, I can maintain my integrity and never have to break vows.

The Vietnam War is starting. When they call my draft number, I refuse to fight and become a conscientious objector, stationed to work in hospital admissions fifty miles from my Philadelphia home. To fulfill my duty, I must leave the Curtis Institute, leave ML, and only come back to the city for weekends to continue my new job at Christ Church.

Working at the hospital, I have plenty of time to explore, especially myself, my true feelings. Slowly I am accepting that while I love women, physically I am drawn to men. I guess I have always known this on some level, and therein lies the battle I have been waging within myself, especially as it regards my relationship with ML. As life moves on, I will have many male lovers, but my heart will always belong to her.

Time passes and ML reluctantly moves on. Even though she now lives in New York City and I don't often see her, she is never out of my thoughts. It is impossible for either of us to imagine a life without the other. Along our journey, our situation causes heartbreak for us both. We have faith that someday the heartbreak will resolve.

She sees me through many crises, she stands by me for decades.

On the occasion of her sixtieth birthday, I write her this note: "There is no way to fasten my head around a love that has already endured forty years, that may not be touched by any living thing. That we knew each other from the start is always the great and unique marvel that does not dim. What an amazing gift is this friendship that has no comparisons. It gives me the true happiness that one gets by opening the first gift under the tree on

Christmas morning and finding out it was the one single thing in life that you really and truly wanted. That's you, darling NuNu! I do so love you always! John."

Six decades into our special relationship, I am slowly dying. NuNu, as I have called my ML ever since her first godson gave her that nickname in the 1970s, is the one I call every morning to say, "I love you, darling." And it is she who answers in kind.

It's now late September 2020. Feeling my time is almost here, I am peaceful. I have no fear of death, never have. Believing I will not see her again, I send one last email: "My dearest NuNu, there is little else but you in my mind and heart these days. I feel so close; love this deep is past words, so I love you past words. Thank you for the gift of you!"

And then, miraculously, I open my eyes and there she is, NuNu, my own private angel, standing by my side to wish me Godspeed on my journey.

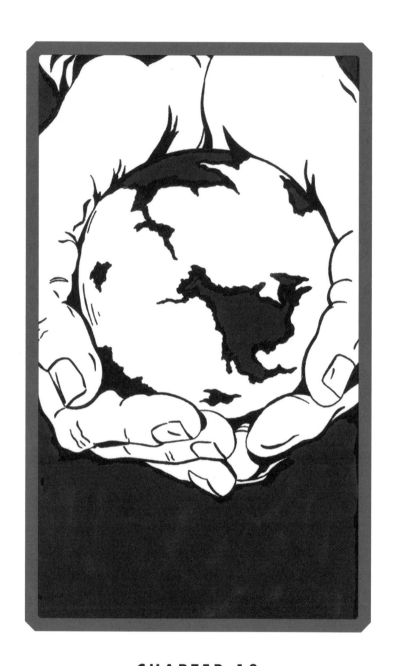

CHAPTER 18

I'm Teaching at Baldwin

n the spring of 1966, during what is to be my last official year at Curtis, I am sure that teaching, not singing, is my future. I have assurances from Glassboro State College in southern New Jersey that it will accept me as a transfer student in the fall. Confident of my next move, I submit my official application while preparing for my Curtis graduation.

Guess what? Just weeks before my senior recital, I am stunned to learn, via a letter from Glassboro, that "with regret" they will not be accepting any transfer students for the fall semester. Now what? Having declared my intentions to Curtis, I have to graduate. Recognizing my plight, it's Curtis to the rescue. Specifically who is my guardian angel, I will never know. The school invites me to come back in the fall as a special student for voice lessons, coaching, and opera workshop, all still under complete scholarship! This is unbelievable. What an extraordinary gesture of kindness, what a gift! I say "yes, thank you" and proceed to round out my good luck for the year ahead with an array of professional singing engagements. I'm in heaven.

And then, just to make things even better, an acquaintance reaches out to me. She is looking for a substitute to take over her classes, teaching general music to grades K–6, in spring of 1967 at the Baldwin School in Bryn Mawr. She's been told that if she can find a suitable substitute, she is welcome to go on tour singing with the Robert Shaw Chorale. I become that "suitable sub," she never returns, and I inherit the job . . . no teachers' college required! How's that for serendipity?

Baldwin's headmistress, Rosamond Cross, is a very progressive thinker who isn't concerned about college degrees. My diploma from Curtis is not the credential normally accepted for this or any other teaching position. It doesn't seem to matter to Miss Cross, who says: "If you want to get a teaching degree, do it for yourself. We are very happy with your work, and a degree will make no difference to us." How extraordinary to encounter this open spirit in the academic world of 1967.

As much as I love teaching at Baldwin and as flexible as they are in allowing me to perform whenever opportunity knocks, I feel this arrangement will not fulfill me in the long term. I just know I need a larger canvas, perhaps even an international one. After eight wonderful years at Baldwin, the time to leave is approaching. I have done everything from eventually chairing the music department to being the 1975 commencement speaker.

When I share my feelings with my mother, she, who lived through the Great Depression, thinks I am out of my mind and says, "Why would you give up security and a good weekly paycheck?" But other options await, and I feel it's almost time for me to move on.

But for the moment, I'm still at Baldwin. I love teaching. What a joy it is to watch the little ones get excited about music. While I have no formal training as a teacher, I do have lots of enthusiasm, and this seems to be a key ingredient in working with children.

During my first year of teaching lower school music at Baldwin, I have a serious problem with a precocious second grader. This very clever child has organized her class into a "family" of chaos. She has assigned a designated role to each of her classmates:

mother, father, sisters, brothers, cousins, addressing each other as "Bover," followed by their first name. She is not only the architect of this chaos but has also assumed the role of the all-powerful "father" figure, calling herself "Bover Caroline." This "family" of twenty "Bovers" appears daily for music class looking to "father" to give the signal for mayhem.

With the permission of the headmistress, I determine that the only way to restore any semblance of order is to remove this ringleader and for a short while, or so I think, have her sit out every daily music class in the office of the headmistress.

What I didn't bargain for was the iron will of this seven-year-old. After two solid weeks, this child doesn't budge from her belligerent position, nor is there any sign of doing so. An apology from her is simply out of the question.

So, I change my strategy. I invite the second grader to be my "teaching assistant," a role that the little tornado accepts and seems to like. To reinforce how important mutual respect is, I tell her that every Friday she will be in charge of the class and, along with her second-grade cohorts, will teach me about the music they love. It works. Phew! I think the unofficial term may be "seat-of-the-pants teaching."

At the end of the school year, the second-grade instigator presents me with a gift, a small book that she thrusts at me with, "Here, this is for you." The book is titled *Thank You for So Many Things*, and the first line reads *"Thank you for being kind and understanding"* and ends with *"Thank you for being You."* In her second-grade handwriting, she has added, "And thank you for such a great year. Wuv, Bover."

A footnote to this story: Thirty years later, I receive a letter from "Bover Caroline," now a lawyer. She has tracked me down to tell me how much she loves classical music and adds, "It all started in that classroom so many years ago. Thank you."

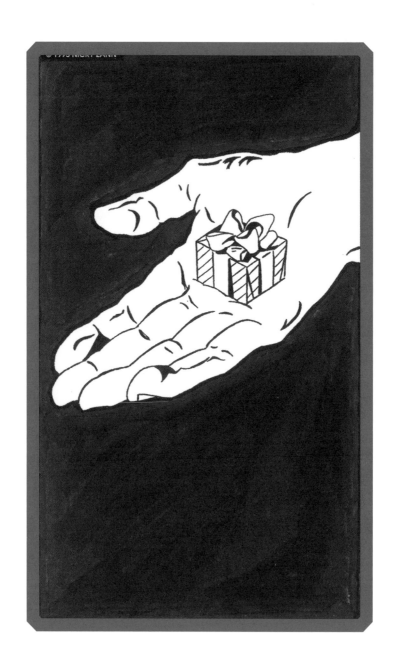

CHAPTER 19

A Person to
Be Remembered

Sometimes people appear briefly in your life and yet make a huge impact. For me, that person is Marcia Sketchley.

An unassuming, former Baldwin student in her late twenties, Marcia really wants to sing and fulfill a lifelong dream of taking voice lessons before it's too late. It's clear she has a severe, debilitating disease, making it extremely difficult for her to even walk.

We start, and Marcia is elated. The first thing we work on is matching a tone. "Hear it, think about it, sing it," I encourage. It's a long and sometimes tedious process. We work week after week, month after month, until she can string notes together and sing a full line of music—many months later, a whole song. She sticks with it, and she succeeds.

I invite her to attend a recital performance I am giving in Philadelphia. She attends with her mother. When she next shows up for her lesson, Marcia tells me that she must stop coming. I ask, "Why this sudden change?" Adding, "You have made such good progress."

She tells me that after attending my recital, she cannot bear the thought of my precious time and talent being spent on her, that she is not worthy of my attention. Her actual words are, "ML, don't waste your time on me."

I carefully but firmly tell her: "Everyone's gift is different. Mine just happens to be singing; that's the gift God gave me." I really need Marcia to understand the depth of my feeling about her, so I continue: "I so admire you! It is I who learn from you at each of our sessions. Weekly you share your enormous gift of courage with me." We continue our lessons.

She doesn't reach her thirtieth birthday, but she does fulfill her dream.

I have never forgotten Marcia Sketchley or what she taught me about humility. To this day, on my desk, I keep a carved piece of scrimshaw that she gifted me all those decades ago. It's a daily reminder of courage, her courage. It's a daily reminder of how lucky I am.

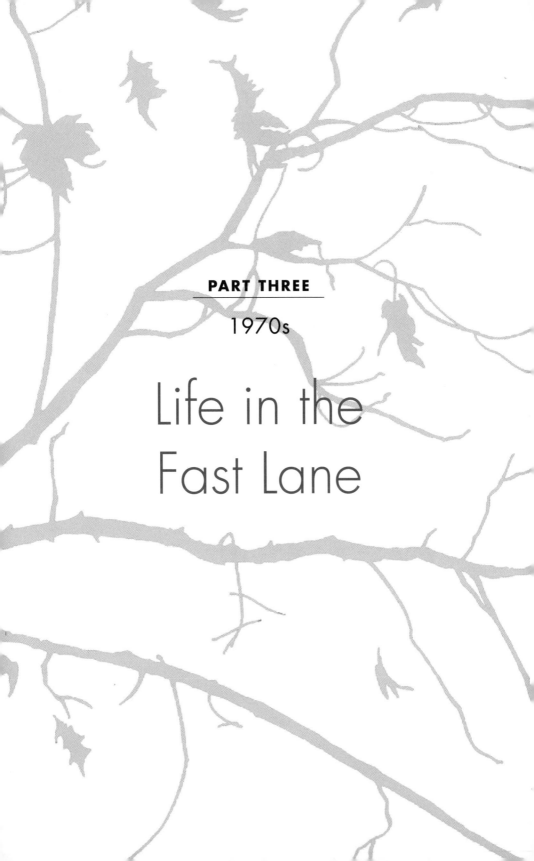

PART THREE

1970s

Life in the Fast Lane

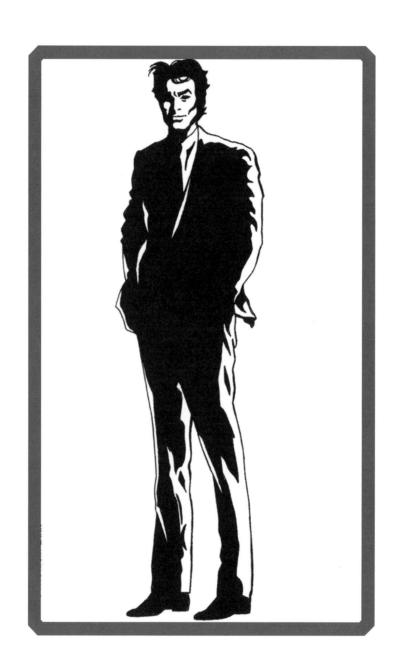

CHAPTER 20

Who Is He?

The date is December 28, 1973, and as I head out to an elegant East Side party, thoughts of Marcia Davenport's novel *East Side West Side* fill my head. Little do I realize that this evening will be a major turning point in my life, one that will leave an indelible imprint that will not be fully realized for another ten years.

When I moved to New York from Philly two years ago, it was to pursue my singing career. Now, I am about to launch my new business, M. L. Falcone, Public Relations, and maybe this holiday gathering will prove helpful. We'll see.

The guests at the posh party are varied and impressive, all there to be seen, and of course to celebrate the opera diva Grace Bumbry's birthday and her new digs. These folks could be a potential treasure trove of contacts, which is precisely the thought of my escort (Grace's accompanist and mine as well) when he invites me to join him. He and I arrive at the party together and quickly go our separate ways.

As I walk into the large living room, all thoughts of business instantly vanish. There, standing with elbow on fireplace and dressed in an Yves Saint Laurent three-piece pin-striped suit, complete with bow tie and red rose bud in the lapel, is the most handsome man I have ever laid eyes on—think Alain Delon. He stops me in my tracks. I silently gasp, my heart thumping wildly, while the romantic phrases of Rachmaninoff's *Symphony No. 2* explode in my head. Plain and simple, I am instantly attracted to him. This is pure animal magnetism.

Who is he? I am determined to find out. I am clearly in his line of sight; he is gazing in my direction.

He walks toward me and makes a point of warmly introducing himself as Nicky Zann. Sparks fly between us. Amazing how his gaze makes me feel like a swan. We chat for a few minutes; then a surprise—his wife, Mary Jo, joins us. A stylishly beautiful blond, we could have been dressed by the same stylist. After chuckling at the similarities of our costumes as well as our names, an immediate rapport is established, and at least from my side, the sparks between her husband and me are dampened, for now.

I learn that Mary Jo and Nicky are both successful artists and friends of Grace's through her then boyfriend. As a power couple in the art world, they are charming, bright, and great fun. We are having a good time and form a trio, breaking off from the rest of the party to enjoy our dinner in the empty library of the apartment. As is fashionable at parties, we vow not to lose touch with each other, a promise we keep.

A beautiful three-way friendship is about to begin, one that will last a lifetime in the most unexpected ways.

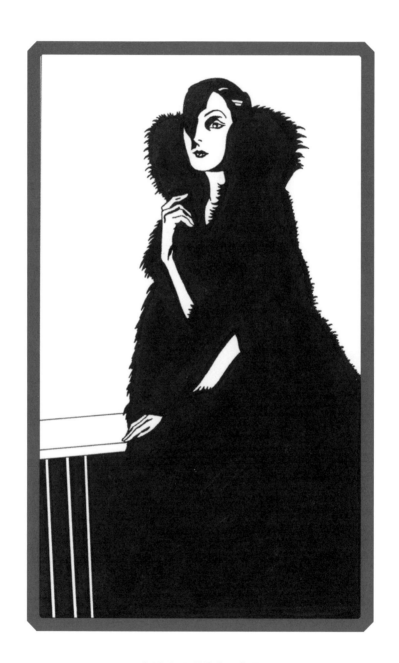

CHAPTER 21

Who Is She?

Another party. My wife, Mary Jo, and I are party animals—well, she definitely is, and I go along. I have stopped counting what number holiday party this is. My buddy has asked us to come and celebrate his opera-singer girlfriend's birthday and inaugurate her new posh East Side high-rise apartment. As these things go, it's pretty boring until I look across the room and my heart stops. Who is she?

Until this moment, I have felt happily married. But suddenly I, Nicky Zann, am overcome with an intense desire to meet this beautiful stranger.

As we near one another, my heart beats faster. What a feeling. It's like love at first sight, which has no place in my life right now. *Des étincelles*—sparks are flying. She introduces herself as ML, and all I can focus on are her deep blue eyes. The spell is broken almost immediately as we are joined by my wife, who takes an immediate liking to her, and an instant friendship is forged among the three of us. Here and now at the end of 1973, I vow to put my desire aside, at least for a time.

Over the next decade, even though being in ML's presence still excites me, I am determined to make my marriage work. While my wife and I are a good team, it's not always easy; I am aware that for her, the grass always seems to be greener somewhere else. By the early 1980s, after fifteen years, I sense our time together is running out. One day she tells me it's over, and I warn her that if she means this and I leave, I am never coming back. She doubts my resolve. I leave—for good. Marriage number two is over, it's amicable, and I am free to pursue the woman of my dreams.

At first ML has a loyalty to my ex-wife and rebuffs most of my advances. But she doesn't completely shut the door. I know in my heart we are meant to be together, and this thought alone propels me to do what I have never had to do with any other woman—I keep trying!

It takes months. She continues to decline almost all of my invitations, always with some polite excuse, but eventually consents to a real date. It is February 28, 1983, and we go to a local Japanese restaurant near her home. After dinner, we return to her apartment for some cuddling and snuggling, and she clearly has an agenda, saying in her most charming tone, "Nick, would you like to spend the night?"

In a split second, I go against my base instinct and say an emphatic "No."

Shocked, she asks, "Why not?"

Carefully, as I have never been clearer about anything in my life, I explain, "I have watched you during the last ten years with your various boyfriends, and your pattern is consistent. When you have finished with an affair or a fling, you graciously tell the poor guy it's over and walk away. That's not for me." As I'm leaving, I add, "If you ever decide you want a real relationship, call me."

Truly, I don't know where I got the strength, because I wanted nothing more than to stay the night. But something deep down told me to call her bluff and make her think about her patterns.

What I said must have resonated, because the next morning she calls and asks me to come over on Friday night for dinner. Assuming she doesn't know how to cook, I bring all the fixings for a steak dinner, cook the entire dinner, and stay for the rest of my life.

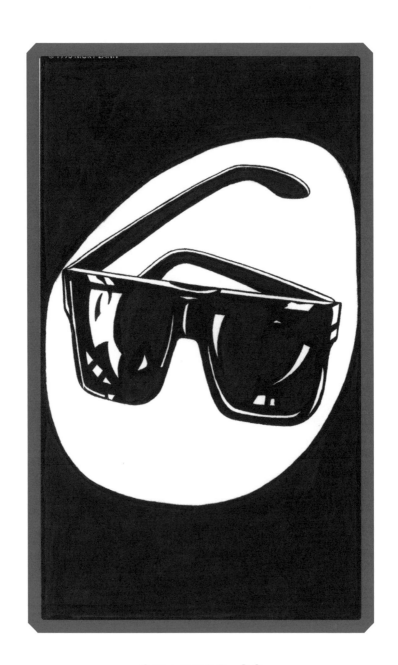

CHAPTER 22

The World-Famous
Pianist Van Cliburn

IT ALWAYS PAYS TO BE 100 PERCENT YOURSELF AND stick to your principles. As I start M. L. Falcone, Public Relations on January 1, 1974, I continue to hold down three jobs, allowing me the freedom to be selective about clients from the very beginning. While continuing to sing professionally and to commute from New York to teach at Baldwin, my fledgling company is definitely gaining traction. There's little room in my life for much else; but if working 24/7 is what it takes to succeed, fine by me. Things are going well, word has spread quickly, and, with no solicitation on my part, prospective clients are calling me. I say yes only to those I believe in . . . maybe not the most economically practical way to start a business, but in my book it's the only recipe for success.

A very high-powered manager, who represented most of the world's great conductors and clearly had been keeping tabs on my business strategy, once said to me: "I don't understand you. You only take on clients in whom you believe. How do you ever expect to make any money?"

Stopping him in his tracks, I answered, "There's one basic difference between us . . . you're greedy and I'm not."

In the category of "only in your dreams," I am told in early 1975 about a major arts organization that is currently pursuing New York's most established public relations firms—that would definitely not be me.

Van Cliburn, the American pianist who set the world on fire in 1958 by winning the first ever Tchaikovsky Piano Competition in Moscow, is often credited with easing the Cold War between the United States and Russia. Now he is looking for a publicist for the piano competition in Fort Worth, Texas, that bears his name, and by extension someone who would also work with him. Three of the most prominent classical music publicists are being wined and dined at New York's finest restaurants by the Texas contingent. When someone tells the Texans about the new kid on the block, the competition officials, exercising due diligence, invite me to the Sheraton Hotel coffee shop, literally for a cup of coffee.

As fate would have it, around the same time, I have taken on an assignment to work on a few US tour dates for a former Cliburn Competition winner. One date is in Detroit where I travel to hear the pianist's recital. The following day my client and I are invited to join a few key Cliburn Competition representatives at a luncheon at the Grosse Point home of Henry and Cristina Ford, where the guest of honor is to be none other than Van Cliburn. This is exciting.

I am the only one in the room that Van doesn't know, and he is inclusive and polite in welcoming me. I, of course, am thrilled just to be in the presence of this giant and enjoy meeting his mother, Rildia Bee. Something clicked that day between me and the Cliburns. Little did I know then how this encounter was going to change my life and take me into the fast lane.

Honey, I am so happy to tell you the account is yours," I announce to ML in a telephone call. "You are the one I want to represent me and my interests. Meet me today at 2:00 p.m. at Orsini's to celebrate."

I enter the elegant New York restaurant carrying two dozen red roses to welcome her. As we sit down to lunch on this chilly March day in 1976, I tell ML that I am a southern boy through and through, as though she can't tell from my thick accent. "I just love southerners, and your spirit is definitely that of a southerner; plus, you have a double first name. And, honey, your family hails from southern Italy, and south is south. We southerners just have to stick together."

Following lunch, off we go to Cartier. I must commemorate the occasion. Perhaps the diamond pin and the rose and yellow gold bracelet will do it. She doesn't see me putting these items on my account, and it isn't until we are back in my limousine that I present them, saying, "Welcome to the family." She is stunned and says she cannot accept the gifts, but I insist.

The more time I spend with ML, the more impressed I am. At one point early on, I think about her romantically, but quickly that notion gives way to thinking about her as the little sister I always wanted. My mother loves her instantly, which is unusual, and sees her as a positive influence on me.

ML, who's eleven years my junior, has no trouble telling me when she thinks I am out of line. This makes me admire her even more and want to shower her with beautiful things—maybe a pair of antique chairs, a Queen Anne chest, a grand piano. She politely sends back the Queen Anne chest to the antique dealer, telling me that enough is enough, and she cannot accept all of this—she says there is a limit, and I have exceeded it!

She also insists that I take back the extra money that I have thrown into her purse, and when I won't, she spends it all on gifts for me and my mother. The note that accompanies the gifts says, "Van, if you persist with this extravagant behavior, I will just keep spending everything that you sneak into my purse on your mother and you." Point taken; lesson learned. Interesting, someone who cannot be bought. Now she is even more intriguing.

I love her company and include her in everything I do. I once told the new owner of Sol Hurok's management company that the only way I could ensure having lunches and dinners with ML on a constant basis was to hire her—maybe it was a bit of an exaggeration, but basically it was true. She is representing my interests and doing a beautiful job. We have a wonderful and productive relationship for seven years. She is faithful to me, and I to her.

Along the way, I have introduced her to all my friends. Almost everyone loves her, but there is one close friend, The Empress, who hates her on sight. ML warned me that it might not be a good match, but I wouldn't listen. The Empress can be ruthless, often instructing her stable of shady characters to be destructive toward her perceived enemies. I begin to fear for ML. My only recourse to protect her is to sever our close ties. And so, after seven wonderful years of close communication and companionship, I stop taking her calls.

ML is very wise and submits her resignation, which I accept, confident that this will protect her. I sense she understands exactly why I am doing this.

Almost a dozen years pass before I see ML again. By the 1990s, The Empress is out of my life, and ML is back and able to handle several difficult situations for me, but will only do it out of friendship—she will not allow me to hire her.

On my deathbed several decades later, she visits me. We laugh and cry, reminiscing about old times. I tell her how much I love her, how proud of her I am. I add, "You have been so special in my life, and I know we'll meet again; we'll be together again." I ask her to make me one last promise: "Please, will you be the one to tell the world about my passing?" She promises she will, and now I peacefully rest, knowing my legacy is in her hands.

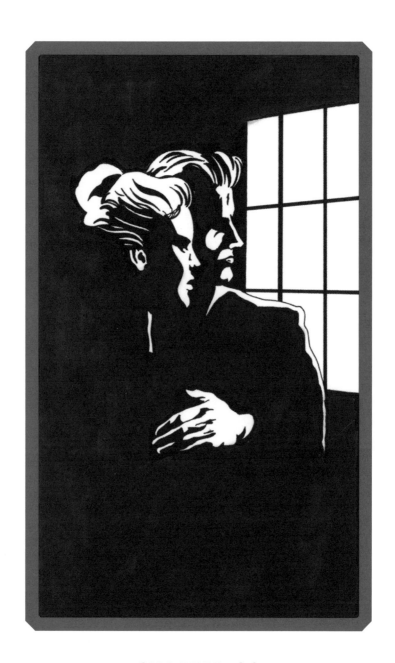

CHAPTER 23

Mother of the World-Famous Pianist

MOTHERS BY NATURE TEND TO BE PROTECTIVE OF their sons. Trying to make sure that Van's overly generous nature didn't get him into trouble, Rildia Bee O'Bryan Cliburn was no exception. Her antennae were up at all times, warning Van about those who would take undue advantage of his good nature. As much as I loved her, I think it's fair to say that her protection went beyond what was reasonable.

For whatever reason, she embraced me from the beginning, probably because I was a no-nonsense person who called it as I saw it, even if my point of view was not always popular with Van. My resolve came from a place of caring and never pandering, not the norm around celebrities. Basically, Rildia Bee and I understood each other. We both wanted what was best for Van.

Sugar," I say to my son, "I really like that young lady; she's different from the rest. She's a good Christian girl. She has humility and really looks out for you."

My son Van dotes on me, and I only want what is best for him. Most people who come into his life want to take advantage of his celebrity and generosity. I watch them, men and women, wanting something and being as sweet as pie to me to curry favor with my son. I really do see it all.

ML is not like that. She has genuine affection for me and I for her, and Van seems to love and trust her.

My son can be impetuous, very often to his own detriment. ML is able to corral his negative impulses and has no trouble speaking up to him when she thinks it's necessary. She is strong, and he has met his match. He listens to her, because he knows truth when he hears it and clearly respects her.

I love this girl. At one point I share my dream with her: "Wouldn't it be a blessing if you could become my daughter-in-law?" I share this with no one but her; it's our secret.

While in my heart, I doubt this will ever happen, I want her to know how I feel. She is only the second person for whom I have ever had these feelings.

Then one day, ML is gone from our lives. I have a pretty good idea who is responsible, but I keep silent.

Twelve years pass, it's 1994, and I am at the end of my life. ML miraculously comes back into our lives just when I need her, just when Van needs her. She supports Van emotionally, and I love her for it. She is there to say goodbye to me, and I feel I can leave this world knowing that my son has someone in his life who will protect him.

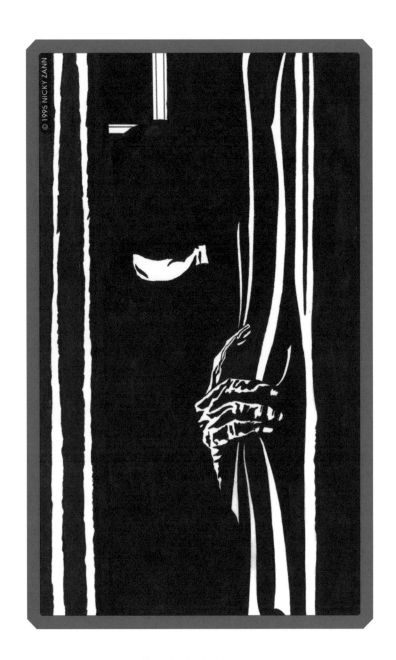

CHAPTER 24

The Empress

I WAS NOW SPENDING A GREAT DEAL OF TIME WITH Van and his friends, most of whom were delightful. However, he had one extremely close friend that I sensed was not going to be an ally. She was powerful and did pretty much what she wanted without ever facing consequences. I repeatedly warned him that singing my praises to her was not a wise idea and that doing so was to tread on dangerous territory. Call it woman's intuition, but I just knew that she had a love for him that she didn't want to share with anyone. He wouldn't listen to reason and insisted that I was wrong." Honey," he would say, "she's just going to love you." I knew the opposite would be true.

While I prefer to see the best in people, sometimes it's difficult. If the eyes are the windows to the soul, then what I saw in the eyes of Van's friend was unsettling to say the least. What made it worse—she knew I saw her, and she found my presence disconcerting. Meeting her in 1977 was the beginning of an odyssey that would not end well.

Never do I travel without my entourage. They love me, I tolerate them. I am a collector of people and possessions. One could say I am prone to excess, but why not? I see it, I want it, I get it.

Celebrities are especially important to my collection. I so enjoy throwing lavish parties to show them off. The more famous, the better.

One of my favorites is Van Cliburn. He is my soulmate. But with him comes his mother Rildia Bee, a bit of an annoyance to me, though I have plenty of people to keep her occupied.

Then one day he brings his friend ML to dinner. She is well dressed, appropriate, and rather quiet. What he sees in her I do not know. What I do know is that she unnerves me. I sense that she sees through me, and I don't like it. This unfamiliar feeling makes me uneasy.

The old adage, "Keep your friends close, keep your enemies closer," comes to mind as I watch her.

My Van is clearly enamored. He raves about her, what a great talent she is. He won't stop. He tells me how she has had a wonderful singing career and now is an extraordinary publicist.

We'll just see about that.

One night, I host a gathering of twenty-five friends at the Waldorf Astoria's Peacock Alley. I invite him to bring her. I hire the house cocktail pianist for the evening. When we get to the dessert course, one of my trusted henchmen asks ML in a commanding voice for all to hear, "You sing, don't you?"

She replies that she used to sing, but no longer does. Whereupon another planted henchman stands behind her, tilts her chair so she has no choice but to stand up—and sing.

I am confident she will fail miserably, given the cruel setup. I do not bargain for a triumph.

As she sings, I watch Van as he watches her, and my blood boils. My sadistic ploy has backfired. He is smitten and proud. I am foiled but undaunted; I will find another way to get rid of her.

It takes me four years. Every time I see a negative news story about me, I point it out to him, saying, "You see, she did this."

Eventually it works, not because he believes me, but because he becomes frightened for her safety. Deep down, he knows what I am capable of.

For seven years, he has had her as one of his closest advisors, confidantes, and friends. She can always get through to him, but one day he just stops taking her calls. I knew I could count on his protective instincts to sever his relationship with her.

Evidently, she senses what is happening and delivers her letter of resignation to him. I can imagine her asking him whether he will tell her the truth someday, to which he would reply, "Maybe someday I can." How quaint.

I have finally succeeded.

Several years pass, and I see ML at a concert and call out to her as if nothing had ever happened. She waves and disappears into the crowd.

A decade later, Van has long stopped communicating with me. But he is back in touch with her. It is she who remains close to him until his death.

Ironically, at his funeral, her small bouquet of white flowers is placed very close to my enormous, heart-shaped rack of red roses, adorned with a huge gold sash declaring my unending love.

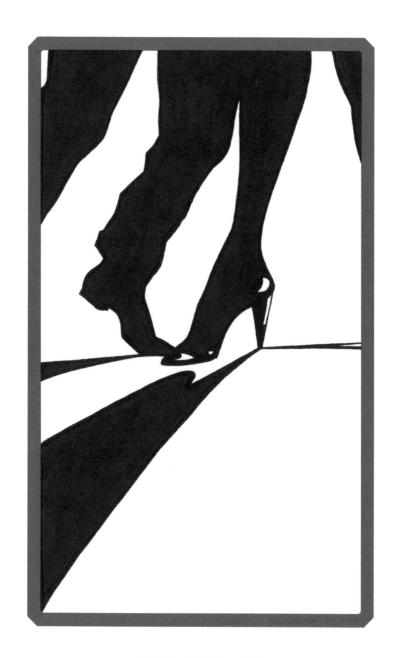

CHAPTER 25

The Older Man

DURING THE EARLY 1970S, BERMUDA WAS A VACATION paradise for me and my close friend Bonnie Lueders, before she married the opera director Frank Corsaro. On one of our first trips, we met two charming men, one of whom was Gus Rego, a well-to-do businessman twenty-five years my senior. Slowly we started a relationship that was to last for the next ten years. While we liked each other, it was more about lust than love, and each of us understood that. When the trysts began, I was still a virgin at age twenty-five, and little did I realize that Gus was the perfect "warm-up act" for what was to become the most important and complete relationship of my life.

Allow me to set the scene: Bermuda, my home, is particularly beautiful this time of year. It's 1970, and the month is May. I frequent a nearby hotel pool; the owners are friends of mine and very accommodating. On this particular day, I am there relaxing with my five-year-old daughter when I hear a voice say, "What beautiful eyes you have." Someone is speaking to my child.

Before I can stop myself, I lower my sunglasses and, staring into the eyes of the lovely stranger, say: "If you think her eyes are special, just take a look at her father's. Hello, my name is Gus." The stranger instantly blushes while her traveling mate, a sexy blond, smiles knowingly.

That's how ML and I meet. I decide to play with fire, a specialty of mine, and invite her and her blond friend Bonnie to my home for dinner that evening. My wife is used to spontaneous entertaining, and these two guests are clearly very nice girls.

Twenty-five years my junior, ML is unmistakably untarnished. The flirtation is delicious, the sparks undeniable, but the real fire has yet to be lit.

A year passes, and she and Bonnie return to the island on vacation. By this time, I am free to pursue her. Again, the sparks fly, and she is full of passion; the combustion is explosive—she has finally been awakened. In that moment, I am very content to think of her as my latest conquest. With several failed marriages under my belt, it's flings with pretty, young ladies visiting Bermuda that I want—not entanglements. The young ladies come, they have fun and leave—perfect!

Let's face it: I'm a wealthy man who loves to play. I really like ML and invite her to be a frequent guest at my Bermuda home overlooking the Atlantic Ocean. I spend an equal amount of time with her in New York City.

It's just the two of us during these interludes. We are hedonists, we are free, there are no strings, and it's fun.

We happily carry on like this for almost a decade. It's a relationship based in the bedroom, and neither of us has expectations of anything more.

She is a serious, hardworking lady; I am a sportsman. I like trophies of all kinds, and she definitely is a trophy.

At the end of our decade together, our long-distance relationship has played itself out. Nothing dramatic, we just stop visiting each other. It's amicable, but it's the end.

Fifteen years pass, with an occasional Christmas card exchanged, and we are now well into the 1990s, my twilight years fast approaching. I have a burning desire to talk to ML, but, not reaching her, I have to settle for leaving a message on her answering machine: "Darling, been thinking so much about you lately. Just want you to know, you are the one that got away, and that is something I regret."

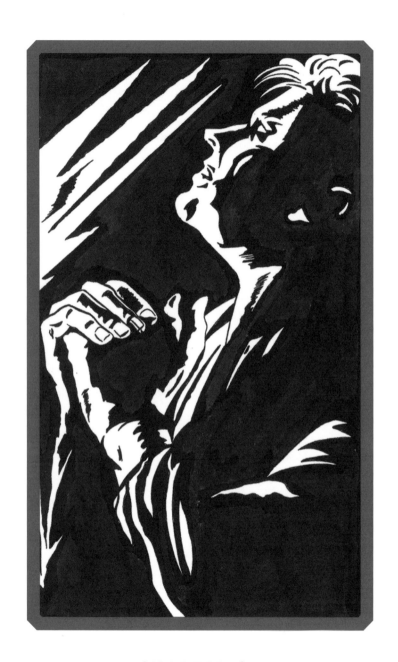

CHAPTER 26

The Priest

UNFINISHED BUSINESS IS OFTEN PAINFUL TO DEAL
with. While John Binsfeld and I were never lovers, we loved
one another deeply. This kind of bond can be threatening
and disconcerting to someone entering a new relationship.
Sometimes the residual impact of the past needs time to
play itself out. And so it was with an extraordinary priest,
Vincent Ioppolo, who just needed a bit of time to realize
that I was not the enemy in his relationship with John.

First and foremost is my love of God. But God help me, as hard
as I try, I can't stop myself from loving temptation too.

My current temptation is a minister of sorts. John Binsfeld is
the minister of music at Philadelphia's historic Christ Church and
has prestige and standing in the community, as do I. He is the
love of my life. Until now, we've been careful to publicly conceal
our feelings for one another, and then the dam breaks. To those
in our respective circles, our forbidden love is now clear.

I lose my composure at a 1971 New Year's Day party. John is
nowhere in sight, but his former girlfriend, ML, for whom he
still has very strong feelings, is about to leave the party as I arrive.
She's aware of what's been going on between us and tells me that
I don't need to worry about her presence in our lives—she will

stay away. She adds, "My care and concern for you both will never change."

Before I can censor myself, I snap back: "Don't you understand? We don't want your care or your concern."

Shocked and visibly hurt by my abrupt response, she leaves without a word.

Five years pass, and I am still guilt-ridden by the way I treated her. I send her an apology, asking for forgiveness. I am no longer a Catholic priest, but have changed my calling to the Episcopal ministry, a better fit for me. And John and I are no longer a couple. Life moves on.

It's now the late 1980s, and I am dying of AIDS in New York City. Drifting in and out of a coma, I hear the rectory phone ringing. My mother, who is caring for me, answers. I pick up the extension next to my bed and recognize the voice of ML, my old-nemesis-now-friend. I listen as she expresses her care and concern for me. Then I speak up, shocking my mother who has not heard my voice in days.

Directly to ML, I whisper, "I love you," and she answers, "Vincent, I love you too." This makes me smile as I drift off.

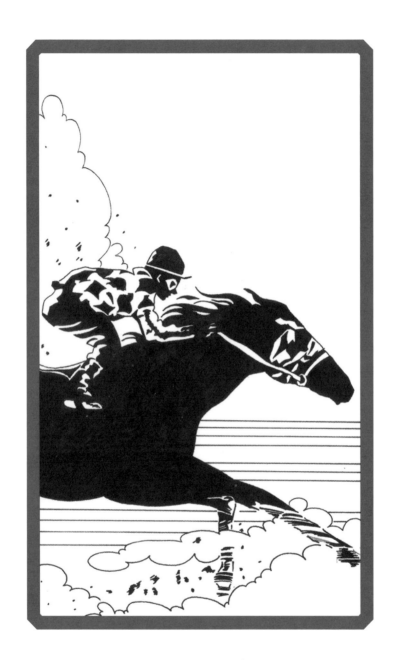

CHAPTER 27

My Big Break

Before the start of my public relations career, I have an eight-year stretch (approximately 1966 to 1974), where performing is my main focus. My first big break in the opera world happens in early 1971. The production of Tchaikovsky's *Queen of Spades*, conducted by Peter Herman Adler, is one of the last of the lavish opera presentations created for television by NET Opera Theater for the National Educational Television network (precursor of the Public Broadcasting Service). The tradition of creating opera in a studio for television audiences started in the early 1950s as the NBC Opera Theatre, with many historic productions, including the world premiere of Menotti's *Amahl and the Night Visitors* and Leontyne Price's legendary performance in Puccini's *Tosca*. Decades later, this tradition is replaced by actual live opera and delayed transmission broadcasts shown on television and in movie theaters from opera houses around the world.

Opportunity knocks in the late 1960s. It's fun to go completely wild and try something new, and so, I do. My audition improvisation of the character—the old, drunk charwoman in Kafka's novella *Metamorphosis*, for the opera version that premieres in Philadelphia—lands me the job and the director's praise.

The opera is a success, and shortly thereafter in 1970, I am invited by the same director, Rhoda Levine, to come to New York and audition for a new NET Opera Theater television presentation of Tchaikovsky's *Queen of Spades*. As I await my turn to audition, I see many major singers, and even some Broadway stars, vying for the mezzo part. It's a long shot, but I know Rhoda believes in me, so, at least I have one friend in my court. The audition goes well, but the conductor has a major reservation—of all things, it's about where I live: Philadelphia and not New York City. Rhoda fights for me, assuring the conductor that I am completely reliable and that geography will never be an issue. Happily, for me, she wins!

At the first rehearsal, the conductor asks, "Do you play piano?"

I respond by saying, "Yes, I play but would never consider myself a pianist."

His answer, "Good!" Handing me the piano score, he adds, "Learn it overnight. As a matter of fact, come in tomorrow with it memorized," which I do.

To my surprise, the instrument is not a piano, but a harpsichord, which I've never played. As I sing the duet accompanying myself and the soprano, I forget to be nervous about singing—all my worry and concentration are on the keyboard.

The entire cast moves from rehearsing in New York City to filming at Boston's WGBH studios. I am dazzled by the opulence of the sets, complete with walls covered by luxurious brocade. I know from earlier fittings in New York that the costumes are equally breathtaking. And I discover that the orchestra is made up of Boston Symphony players, so, I guess you might consider this my harpsichord debut with the Boston Symphony. If that isn't enough glitter, the legendary mezzo-soprano Jennie Tourel has been cast as the old Countess, luxury casting to be sure. This is historic, and I am part of it—pinch me!

Everything is going well, and I seem to be fitting in just fine. One day, I get an unexpected compliment from the conductor. Each morning, preparing for the day by rising early and bracing for the extremely brisk New England weather, I bundle up and walk the mile from the hotel to the studios, while my colleagues are chauffeured. Evidently, the conductor has been watching me do this and comments to my fellow cast members how impressed he is. For me, it's simply about clearing my head and feeling invigorated before being cooped up (as exciting as it is) in a studio for hours—and besides, I tend to get carsick in over-heated cars and don't want to chance it.

I am twenty-five years old, the opera airs nationally in January 1971, and my singing career is on its way.

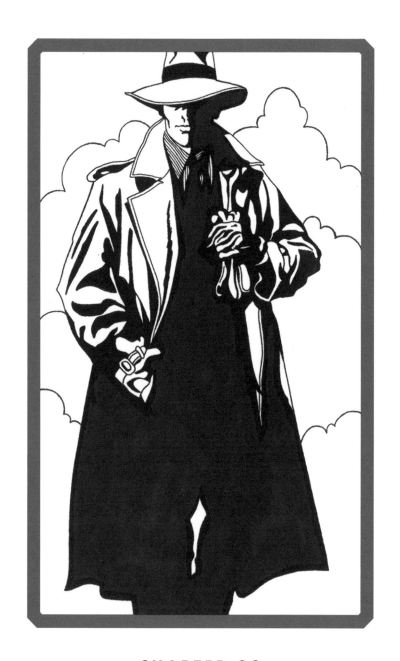

CHAPTER 28

The Maverick
Opera Director

I WILL FOREVER BE GRATEFUL TO MY WONDERFUL
friends, the brilliant maverick director Frank Corsaro and
his very special and multitalented wife, Bonnie Lueders, for
keeping watch over me when I first moved to New York City
in 1971. Frank was one of America's foremost stage directors of opera (legendary productions of the 1960s, '70s,
and '80s at New York City Opera) and theater (among his
many Broadway productions were *Night of the Iguana* with
Bette Davis and *Baby Want a Kiss* with his close friends
Paul Newman and Joanne Woodward); plus, he was artistic director of the famed Actors Studio. Bonnie did everything from opera singer to Broadway star to masterful
flower designer to creator of a line of cookies known as
Bonnie's Best.

Our close relationship lasted more than five decades,
and in those early days, thanks to their generous hospi-
tality, I met numerous influential people, many of whom
became friends, colleagues, and allies. Bonnie, Frank,
and their son, Andrew, my godson who gave me the nickname NuNu, were my New York "family." Bonnie and Frank
stayed married but went their separate ways, and I continued to maintain strong bonds with both. As fate would

have it, I kept watch over Bonnie during the final six months of her life until she died in 2016. Frank's death, ironically from Lewy body dementia, came a year later, giving closure to a complicated karmic circle. It makes me happy that godson Andrew Corsaro and his wife, Denise, along with their two sons, continue to be part of my extended "family."

My life is all about drama. At forty-nine, I, the confirmed bachelor Frank Corsaro, have just proposed to the beautiful blond opera singer Mary Cross Lueders, known to all as Bonnie. Our wedding date is set for May 1971, just before I am scheduled to direct the world premiere of the opera *Summer and Smoke*, based on Tennessee Williams's play. To celebrate our engagement, my fiancée, Bonnie, has invited her dearest friend and college roommate, ML, who is to be our maid of honor, to join us in New York.

What comes to mind as ML and I meet for the first time? "You're the one who cooks a dynamite lasagna. How about cooking up a batch for me and a few of my friends?"

Her reply, "Sure, I'd be happy to."

And so, joining us on that winter evening for the divine lasagna feast are my *Summer and Smoke* pals: the composer Lee Hoiby, the librettist/playwright Lanford Wilson, and music publisher Bob Holton. Somewhere toward the end of dinner, Lanford, staring at ML says, "You look exactly the way I envision one of the characters in our opera. Do you sing?"

"Yes," is her reply, whereupon Lee goes to the nearby piano and says, "Just sing this for me." Too shocked and surprised to protest, ML sings and is hired on the spot.

Following the May wedding, ML joins my new bride (who is also in the *Summer and Smoke* cast) and me, plus everyone else who was at the lasagna feast, and we all reunite in Saint Paul, Minnesota, for the opera's world premiere.

Just a short postscript, which I cannot resist: The opera is a resounding success with audiences and critics. In fact, it's so successful that my friend Tennessee Williams, who is with us, proclaims at the after party that he prefers the opera to his play.

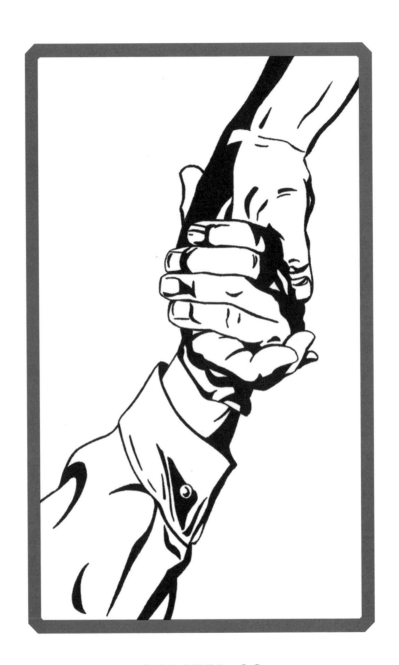

CHAPTER 29

Lifelong Friend, MB

THE SAINT PAUL OPERA ENRICHED THE LIVES OF MANY singers, allowing us to spread our wings as performers, and in my case, presenting me with a unique window of opportunity to look into my future profession. It is where I met my friend Mary Beth Peil (MB), who remains a treasured confidante more than fifty years later. Following her career as an opera singer, Mary Beth went on to become an Obie Award–winning, two-time Tony Award–nominated actress who is as comfortable in musical theater as she is in plays, on television, or in movies. You might know her as Yul Brynner's last Anna in *The King and I*, or perhaps Grams in *Dawson's Creek* or Jackie in *The Good Wife*. Now in her eighties, she continues to be a working actor in constant demand.

t's 1971 and in Saint Paul, Minnesota, the world premiere opera *Summer and Smoke* is about to garner worldwide attention. I have been cast as the leading lady, Alma, and a group of both well-established and up-and-coming artists fill out the opera company roster. All the artists care about one another and rejoice in being part of this special summer repertory "family."

Among the "family" members is ML. We bond immediately and become lifelong friends—Mary Beth and Mary Lou, known to all as MB and ML.

Since *Summer and Smoke* is such a huge success, even receiving positive comments from the playwright himself, the Saint Paul Opera decides on a reprise the following summer. ML and I decide to rent a house together, the Seymour house on glorious Summit Avenue. We christen our favorite spot in the house the "Seymour Kitchen," and later affix that name to anyplace in the world where we happen to find ourselves together sharing dreams. In our Seymour Kitchen, we laugh and we cry, and we imagine our futures. And when our dreams become reality, which they often do, new dreams are created. ML and I have now been doing this for more than fifty years.

In the summer of 1972, we are free most mornings, with plenty of time to daydream and visualize over our beloved Seymour Kitchen coffeepot.

ML is restless, sure there is a third act for her, if only she can find it. Her first and second careers, performing and teaching, are wonderful, but she keeps insisting something is missing. She's always probing for what she is meant to do. Often, she references the fact that, while she loves singing, she doesn't really need to sing, unlike the rest of us. She is constantly making the distinction between want and need. She tells me, "To have a career as a performer, *want* is never enough; the field is flooded with people who want it and think it's fun. You must *need* to perform more than anything, and honestly, MB, I don't need it. I do need to communicate, but it doesn't have to be through singing. There must be something out there, and one of these days I'll find it or it will find me."

Then one morning, something quite unusual occurs—perhaps it's a preview of coming attractions. Our opera company's general manager calls ML, who is chatting with me in our Seymour Kitchen. He is in a panic, because there's a major photo shoot scheduled that afternoon, and the national public relations rep is missing in action. He needs someone to organize and run the shoot. Will ML bail him out and do it?

Interesting that he would call her out of the blue, but he knows what we all have realized. Even though she's younger than the rest of us, she is the real grownup in the company, and she speaks with a voice of authority and confidence that everyone recognizes. She's a leader.

The look on her face when she returns from that shoot is euphoric, transformed. A seed has been planted. She knows it, the general manager knows it, and I know it.

Important ideas need space and time to grow. A year goes by, and in the summer of 1973, another light bulb moment happens, this time at a Saint Paul Opera donors cocktail party.

The conversation at this party is about the company's image. ML's imagination is piqued, and she holds court on the subject. When asked if she is serious, she quips: "Of course not. I was just having fun playing with the concept," but quickly adds, "I could be serious." She confides in me that maybe this is the platform she has been looking for. Perhaps organizing last summer's photo shoot for the opera was not an isolated event, perhaps it was a sign.

She muses: "Maybe I could talk about a field that I love and know a lot about and get paid for it. This is certainly worth looking into."

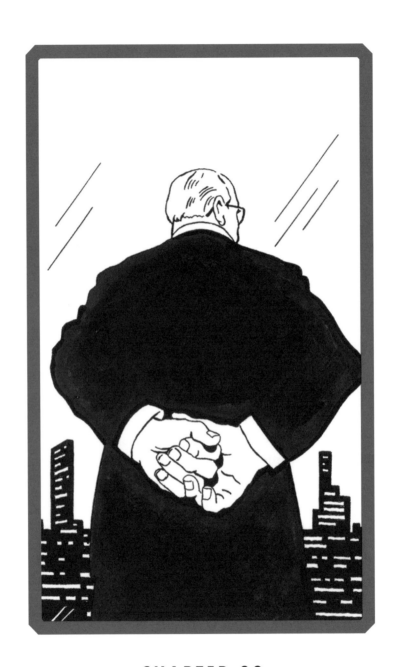

CHAPTER 30

Opera Company
General Manager

EVERYTHING WAS MOVING FAST, AND MY HEART AND head were spinning with possibilities, always a good sign. Just maybe I was onto something, and my friend Mary Beth Peil saw it too. What I have always trusted is my gut; if it says yes, I just know I can do it. I began to feel the inner stirring—the need to wake up excited and challenged every morning—about to be fulfilled. What I have always known is that hard work is a requirement for anything worthwhile, and that is something I have never been afraid of. I was getting closer, closer to finding my true path, closer to having that shot at being the best.

Saint Paul Opera General Manager George Schaefer was a visionary who was about to offer me the chance of a lifetime. As you will discover, it is he who took a leap of faith that made my public relations career real.

My company was launched officially in 1974, and within a month I had a stable of clients. I think the business grew quickly for two reasons: The artists knew I was one of them and trusted that I understood them, and I championed exceptional talent. My motto then as now: Integrity is the key ingredient—without it, you have nothing.

What became clear about a year into this new business was that I would soon be retiring—first from teaching (1975) and then from singing (1977, appropriately with a Verdi *Requiem* in Flint, Michigan). And that's exactly the way it went.

My opera company in Minnesota is my "family," and as general manager, I want to be surrounded by people I like. I like ML, who has sung with us for three seasons. I now invite her to join us for a fourth, telling her, "I love you and love having you as part of this company, but I hate your voice." She accepts my offer and signs another contract, seemingly unfazed by my comment—not a typical singer's reaction.

The phone rings in mid-October 1973, and it is ML telling me that she has been thinking about her future and wonders if, next summer in her free time, she could volunteer in our public relations department. What sparked this, she says, is the little taste of public relations that she got more than a year ago while doing me the favor of running a company photo shoot. She adds, "I have been thinking about it ever since. Now I would love to explore how things work behind the scenes. I have begun to realize that what happens off stage might be as interesting and possibly as powerful as what happens on stage."

Having seen her organizational skills in action, I tell her that I have some other thoughts that I would like to share with her next month over dinner in New York.

When we meet, we talk for six hours about the image of my company. Her ideas are original and exciting.

I always trust my instincts, so, I end our dinner by saying, "Forget about being a volunteer, I want you to be the national and international press rep for the company." As her jaw drops,

I explain, "We would be one client and not a full-time employer, and if you want to start a real business in public relations, you will have to find others who might want your services."

Stunned, she takes a deep breath and says: "I have two major concerns. The first is that I recently moved to New York and don't want to live in Minnesota." That one is easy to solve. I tell her that she needs to be in New York City, where most of the journalists she will be cultivating are based.

She follows with her second concern: "I don't know the first thing about public relations." To this, I have a simple and direct answer: "I have been watching you for several seasons and know you love challenges. Just say yes and go figure it out."

We become her first client.

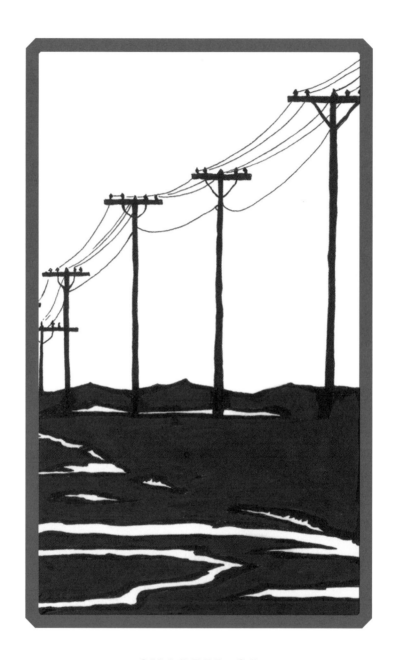

CHAPTER 31

Doyenne of Publicists

AS I ENTERED THE WORLD OF PUBLIC RELATIONS AT age twenty-eight, the old guard, all of whom were considerably older than I, were not too welcoming. As I had never worked in the field, much less apprenticed to a master publicist as they all had, I think perhaps my colleagues perceived me as a young upstart or, worse, an interloper.

There was one person, however, who was secure enough to want to at least find out about this neophyte. That person was Alix Williamson, a thoroughly seasoned and formidable pro, whom I admired and grew to love. She was one of a kind, from the "old world" school of publicists, a flack (I still hate that term), as they were once called.

In her day, Alix was ablaze with public relations ideas and stunts. Among her many celebrated clients was Maria von Trapp. It was Alix who convinced and helped the Baroness to write her memoir, *The Story of the Trapp Family Singers*, later adapted as the Broadway musical *The Sound of Music*—and we all know what became of that genius idea. Thank you, Alix!

Who is this newcomer M. L. Falcone? For years, about six of us in the classical music public relations business have been dominating the market. We are all around the same vintage, roughly in our fifties, and have been doing this for a very long time. We all started from the bottom and worked our way up over the years.

This twentysomething, who has never worked in the field, just started her own shop out of the blue. She interests me. I am curious.

One particularly mean-spirited colleague among us has called her a ruthless bitch—I guess ML landed a client she wanted. Others say she is knowledgeable and quite nice. I will just have to see for myself. What I do know about her is, having never worked in this field, she already has an impressive clientele.

I invite her to lunch, and we have a wonderful time. Toward the end of lunch, I ask bluntly, as is my way: "So, everyone says you are nice. Are you?"

She smiles and answers, "Well, Alix, I guess we will just have to have many more lunches together so that you can decide for yourself."

We become good friends, and over the years I make the claim that she is the best in the business. After me, of course.

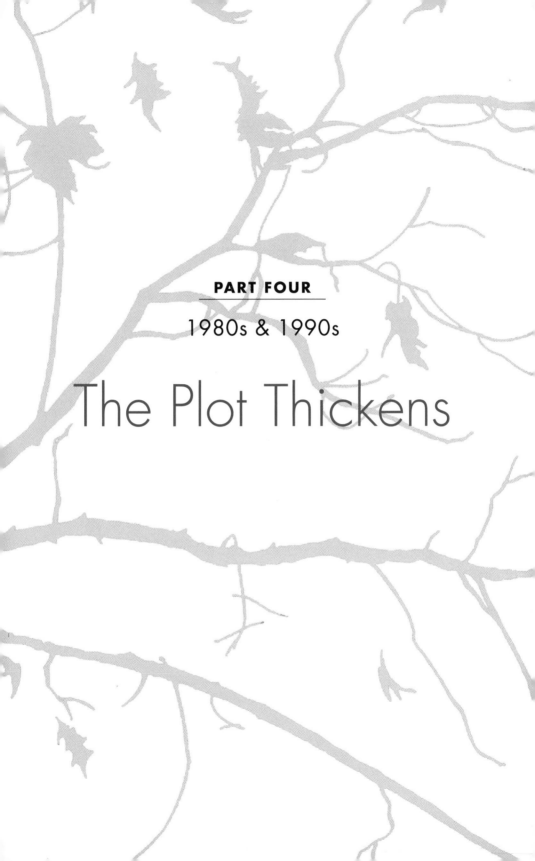

PART FOUR

1980s & 1990s

The Plot Thickens

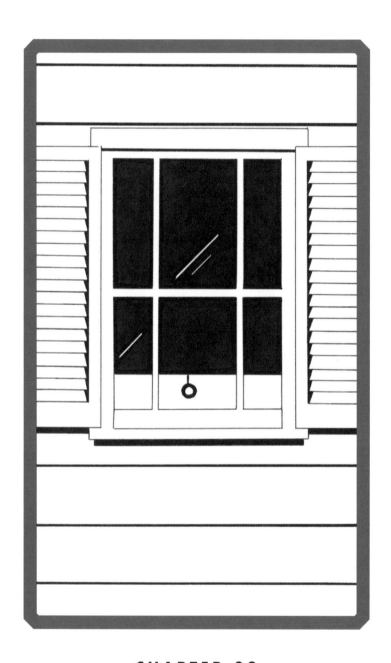

CHAPTER 32

The Soviet Pianist Defects

IN GENERAL, I HAVE FOUND IT WISE TO KEEP WORK and romantic entanglements separate. And with very little room for personal relationships during the 1970s, the issue never surfaced. During the late seventies, I sensed some interest beyond our business dealings from the powerhouse pianist Alexander Toradze, known to all as Lexo. I viewed it as a harmless flirtation, but little did I realize where it would lead, much less the complications it would pose a few short years later.

It's the closing ceremony of the 1977 Van Cliburn International Piano Competition in Texas, and my eyes follow ML as she stage-directs the finalists, myself included. Boy, is she strong and authoritative, a real turn-on! I find out she's older than I am, but no matter, she is hot.

The Cold War continues to rage between the United States and the Soviet Union. As the silver medalist of this competition, I am permitted, thanks to Van Cliburn's standing as a hero in the Soviet Union, to travel from Moscow to the United States for concerts arranged by the competition, of course always with a KGB "chaperone." ML, who is based in New York City, helps me and the other competition winners with publicity surrounding these concerts. Seeing her again on a trip to New York, the electricity that I sensed at that 1977 valedictory ceremony is still alive, and she seems to notice me too.

As we spend time together, the attraction between us gradually blossoms and finally cannot be contained.

ML is very clever and careful, as she does not want to put me in jeopardy, and there is always the omnipresent "chaperone" to contend with. She finds out what the KGB "chaperone" is interested in and then arranges outings for him to enjoy some of the wonders of New York City. She organizes it so that he will be gone for hours, leaving us time for passionate trysts. These encounters, which I admit started with thoughts of her helping my career, lead to genuine love, a love that endures and sustains through several years. Even during the years I cannot be with her, we remain close, communicating through very careful letter writing.

Then comes April in Paris, 1982. I find out during a March concert tour in Yugoslavia that I have been engaged for a last-minute orchestral performance at the end of April at Salle Pleyel. I immediately write to ML and plead with her to join me in Paris for a few romantic days together.

I know she really wants to come, but I also know she is questioning her decision. The Soviet contingent in Paris will be strong, because I am Georgian and the guest conductor for my performance with the Orchestre National de France is Russian. We will be surrounded by "chaperones." It has been almost three years since I have seen ML. Will she be as I last remember her? More important, will she even come?

She arrives on a sleepy Parisienne Sunday and comes directly to my hotel room from the airport. When I open the door, we just stand gazing at one another. Then, following a long wordless embrace, the rediscovery starts, lasting hours, making up for three years of lost time.

Following my performance of the Prokofiev *Second Piano Concerto*, special because ML is with me, I find a way to extend my Paris stay by a few days so that we can enjoy April in Paris together.

A month later, she writes: "We had but a few moments, which no one can ever take from us. Love that is shared so completely needs only the beauty of those moments to sustain a lifetime: Most never experience even one moment of pure truth in love."

A year passes, and I am more resolved than ever to leave the Soviet Union for good, but that also means leaving behind my beloved family in Georgia. With the help of some well-placed American friends, I hatch a plan to defect. With luck, I will know freedom by summer's end. Only the friends who are aiding me know my plan.

My defection is planned for the time I am in Madrid to perform with the Bolshoi Orchestra. It is September 1, 1983, and I hide under blankets, lying on the floor of the back seat of a rental car driven by my dear, well-connected American "family." We glide through the gates of the American Embassy—we have made it, and I can breathe again. I ask for and receive asylum—freedom at last, thank you, United States of America! The plan is for me to come to the States via Rome.

After landing in Rome, I call ML. She gasps at my news, clearly startled, but happy that I have made it to safety. I tell her that she is one of the reasons I needed to be free. She explains that she is now in a serious relationship and that my defection, while thrilling, comes as a shock. Not surprisingly, she is confused. I tell her calmly that I am coming to New York in October, and I will fight for her.

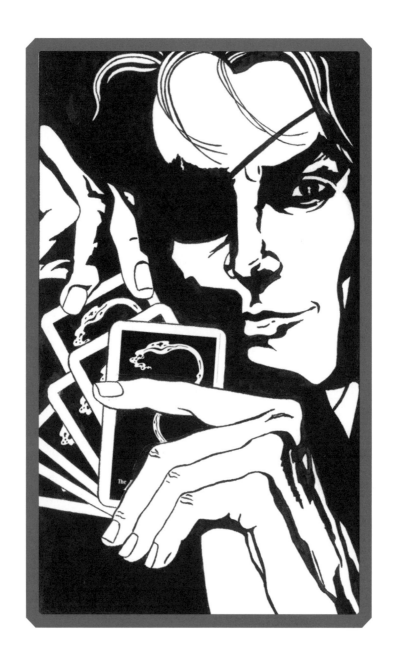

CHAPTER 33

NZ in Love

ROMANCE IN THE 1970S WAS IN SHORT SUPPLY, AND by age thirty-eight, I was resigned to the distinct possibility of being a solo act for the rest of my life. I'd almost given up hope of finding love, of finding that special life partner—someone with whom I could laugh, cry, and share. Enter for the second time my gorgeous, charming, and oh-so-talented friend, Nicky Zann.

It's 1983 and Nicky, having just amicably divorced his wife, Mary Jo, is persistent about pursuing me. The early sparks of ten years ago were never completely extinguished. Truth: While Nicky was married, the flirtations were flattering. Now that he is actually free, I am frightened of a real relationship.

I confess that my actions during the early days of our courtship were nothing short of horrible. Nicky would appear at my Fifty-Seventh Street office in his black leather jumpsuit to present me with one red rose. My response: a polite "thank you" before literally shutting the door in his face. He would return, this time disguising himself in a three-piece tweed suit and horn-rimmed glasses, hoping that this costume and a red rose would turn the key. I rebuffed him and his dinner invitations, and often canceled

lunch plans. In short, I was afraid that we would not be a
compatible duo—our lifestyles were just too different, or so
I thought. Nicky had allowed me, and most everyone else in
his sphere, to see only his wild, fun-loving, public persona.
I had no idea of the depth that lay in wait.

As it turns out, Nicky was much wiser than I. He saw from
the beginning what I didn't . . .

Ten years and one amicable divorce later, ML and I are now free
to be a couple. I knew from the moment I saw her all those
years ago, she was my soulmate.

It's the end of February 1983, and the beginning of the best
years of my life. Having spent several months pursuing her, she
finally says yes to my dinner invitation and realizes during our
date that I am playing for keeps and not for kicks. This I make
very clear when I turn down her invitation to spend our first-
date night in her bed. I would have loved to accept, but I am
determined to have a lasting relationship with her. I know we are
meant to be together, to weather life's joys and hardships.

When I return a few days later for a second date, our life
together begins. There are more highs than either of us could have
anticipated. There are also some stormy moments. I know I am a
wild card, a free spirit, always having been allowed to do exactly
what I want. Most of the time it works out well, but I admit to
sometimes going over the top, and I know these occasions make
her very uncomfortable.

ML is a woman of untamed passion. Everyone has seen this
passion in her work, but rarely, she tells me, has it revealed itself
in her personal life. Some refer to her as the "Ice Princess," and
those are the very people who are shocked to see that we are an
item. It's amazing to see how many suitors appear when it looks

like I am permanently on the scene, almost as if they are seeing her for the first time. Sorry, fellas, too late.

Yet, with all our happiness and passion, we have an unsettling moment of real doubt early on. During the late summer of 1983, about six months into our relationship, a former boyfriend, a Soviet Georgian pianist, defects to the United States, determined to have his lady back. Confronted by this new reality and not having seen him in over a year, ML is confused and does not know what she feels. She must see if the old feelings are alive—without doing this, doubt will always exist.

Were it anyone else, I would simply say, "Goodbye, finito, I don't need this. Why should I stick around to possibly be dumped?" Initially I understand where she is coming from, but my patient attitude doesn't last. After some careful soul searching, I stay around for the outcome, because I have faith that we are meant to be life partners and that she too will realize this.

She goes, she sees him, and she knows—we are meant to be.

What a couple we are! I ask her many times to marry me. Her answer is always the same, "Why let a piece of paper spoil perfection? Let's just enjoy being together without strings." I go along. It is working, and we are a power couple in many ways. She is at the top of her public relations game, respected and trusted by all. I used to think that my days as a 1950s rocker were the highlight of my career. Now as a caricaturist/illustrator/cartoonist, I am in demand, and my work is showing up everywhere, from television to museum collections. I even plan to paint—there's so much I want to say on canvas.

ML and I seem to be a matched set. For the next thirty-seven years, people refer to us as "the golden couple, the fun couple, the couple you can count on."

ML is the love of my life.

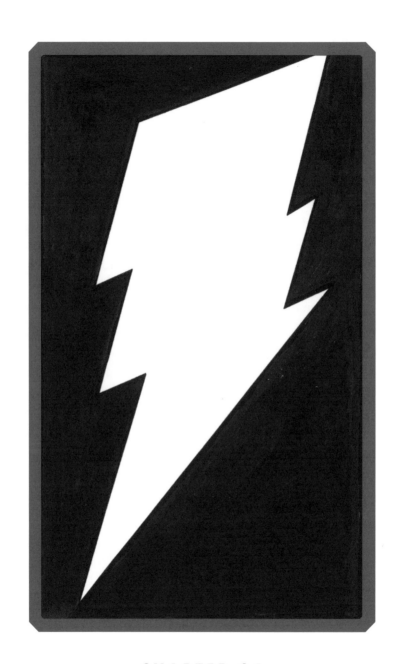

CHAPTER 34

I Find My Soulmate

When Nicky Zann first crossed my path in late 1973, the initial attraction between us was unmistakable. Time for personal relationships was scarce, so it's lucky for me that he was married and didn't seriously surface again in my life until 1983, after his divorce was finalized. Perfect timing. My business has had a ten-year running start. Now I can afford to give in to romance and spend time exploring and enjoying its pleasures.

This second time around, I am constantly making myself unavailable with all kinds of excuses—giving Nicky a very hard time and being quite dreadful. What's wrong with me? I'm scared. My excuse: He is too wild, he won't fit into my serious, slightly stuffy world.

I am both right and wrong. Initially he is wild—a true maverick, a free spirit, always doing and saying exactly what he wants, even when it's not appropriate. For instance, on one of our first dates, I take him to a concert conducted by a musician I represent. At intermission, he comments that the conductor looks lonely up there bowing all by himself; so perhaps at the end of the concert, he will stand up in his seventh-row center seat and bow back to the conductor, just to keep him company. While I think this is a joke, I also know that Nicky is perfectly capable of doing it.

Needless to say, the rest of the concert is ruined for me as I am consumed with worry—will he or will he not embarrass me?

While I harbor occasional doubts about us, my stronger instinct is to give this relationship a real shot—without marriage! After all, he has had two marriages already (one annulment, one divorce). Let's just see where this will go.

The relationship flows and grows stronger and deeper over the next thirty-seven years. We are in tune with each other and completely in love.

He is an artist and with that comes temperament—an irresistible hook for me. He is afraid of no one. He treats the janitor with precisely the same respect and dignity that he treats an international diplomat. There is no pretense, he is 100 percent who he is. Adults love him, children love him, animals love him—and I am completely in love with him.

Saying "yes" to our first date back in 1983 gave me a chance to realize what he always knew—we were soulmates.

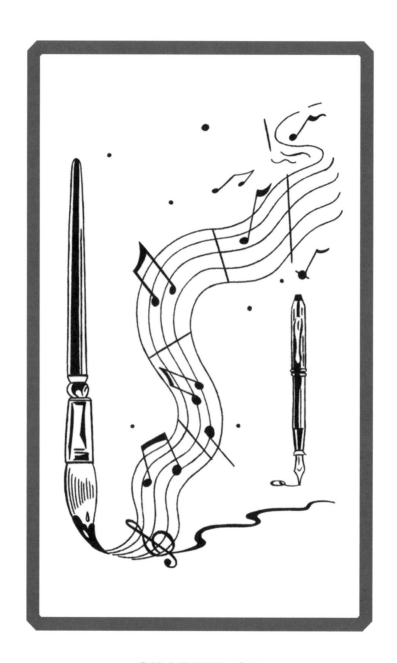

CHAPTER 35

Sextet of Clients

WHEN I LEFT PERFORMING, I NEVER LOOKED BACK. Fulfillment now came from being behind the scenes, and in many ways it was a greater thrill and a better fit than being in the spotlight. What I sensed was that my contributions counted. There were important lessons to be learned, and those lessons were often symbiotic. Over my public relations career, I have been associated with dozens of artists and institutions, many of them remaining with me between fifteen and forty years, a track record of which I am very proud. The longevity of these relationships allowed us to build together. The artists and I never signed contracts, as I felt a handshake was just as binding and honorable. In today's society, I might not opt to work that way, but fifty years ago, it was my path of choice, and it served me well.

The artists highlighted in this chapter represent a microcosm of the music business I serve, as well as important moments of clarity. Along the way I worked with many great artists, and since I don't want to bore you with a shopping list, suffice it to say that in addition to those named in this chapter and those referenced throughout other chapters, my early client list started with the Philadelphia Orchestra and expanded to the Chicago Symphony, Carnegie Hall,

New York Philharmonic, Vienna Philharmonic, Los Angeles Philharmonic, Switzerland's Lucerne Festival, Birgit Nilsson Foundation, Jean-Pierre Rampal, Isaac Stern, Sir Georg Solti, Eugenia Zukerman, Jean-Yves Thibaudet, Gustavo Dudamel, Jaap van Zweden, André Previn, and James Taylor. Having never solicited a client, it's a miracle that I got to represent everyone with whom I ever dreamed of working.

As you may sense from the sample vignettes, guiding and shaping the careers of artists for me is a form of caregiving/caretaking in its broadest sense.

THE DARING VIOLINIST

When I walk into ML's office, the first thing I say is, "I hate ass-kissers."

Without missing a beat, she replies, "Thank goodness, so do I."

I am nineteen years old and from that moment on, I know that I can trust her to guide my career, a career destined to shatter the image of the traditional violinist. Against all odds, she encourages me to be 100 percent who I am, from the way I dress—wearing elegant jumpsuits on stage instead of gowns—to passionately making music without a filter, letting it flow from my heart and soul.

Along the way she does more than guide my career, she helps save my life. It's an early October day in the 1990s, and my career is booming. ML has already orchestrated a feature on CBS's *60 Minutes*, and the world not only knows who I am, it is following my every move. My violin playing is winning people over from all walks of life, and classical music is becoming hip. From the outside looking in, I have it all—all but someone to love who loves me back. An affair of the heart has gone so wrong that the only thing I see is hopelessness and no way forward. A friend is with me at my apartment when I lift a loaded derringer to my head, pull the trigger and, as fate would have it, the gun jams. My freaked-out friend immediately calls ML, who is on my doorstep within ten minutes. She removes the weapon, reassuring me that everything is going to be all right.

Along with a few close friends, she develops a strategy to get rid of the gun and to get me help.

It's always about strategy with ML, whether it's the stuff that careers are made of or, as in this case, dealing with the police. At this moment, ML is determined to get the gun out of the house, no matter what. She phones the local police precinct and, when they arrive, tells them that she has found this "thing" and doesn't know if it's real or a toy. She continues by saying that her friend (that would be me) is ill with the flu in the other room. And, by the way, does New York City still have the amnesty program that empowers the police to remove a weapon from the premises, no questions asked?

The answer: They will take the gun, but have to run it through ballistics to make sure it doesn't have a history. Mercifully, it doesn't. It had been given to me by a well-intentioned friend at a time when I was being hounded and stalked (the price of celebrity), and the friend thought I should be able to protect myself. No more guns!

ML and I, Nadja Salerno-Sonnenberg, work together for thirty wonderful years. After my beloved grandmother, she is my guardian angel.

THE PHILANTHROPIST

In the early 1980s, an attractive, professional young woman catches my attention as someone I would like to work with on my awards program, the Avery Fisher Artist Program at Lincoln Center.

ML and I develop a wonderful relationship, and we truly value each other's opinions and advice. For example, I advise her to always keep notes on important discussions, even if she is not likely to ever refer to them again. "It is prudent to keep written proof," I tell her, "as everyone thinks they will remember details, but as time passes, so do the details." ML often references how valuable this advice is.

In return, she is a great resource for me. One day, I need some advice and call ML to ask what she might know about a certain well-known musical organization. She succinctly and politely replies that their work and musical reputation are excellent. When I probe further about their fiscal responsibility, she tells me: "After working with them for a few years, they decided that I was not getting them enough attention and terminated our relationship. That was fine and fair, but they owed me several thousand dollars for services already rendered. After invoicing them for a full year, I finally gave up and chalked it up to a loss." She also tells me that she knows of other similar instances but, since she does not know those details firsthand, she is not comfortable commenting on the experiences of others.

Well, the very next morning, her phone rings, and it is the head of the musical organization in question telling her the exact amount they owe her, adding that they are prepared to pay her, after ten years!

She replies that she would prefer they pay someone who currently needs the money—she wrote it off a long time ago.

His reply, "Don't you realize that you have single-handedly prevented us from getting a major gift from Avery Fisher?"

Her reply, "Maybe next time you think someone is too insignificant to be compensated for services rendered, you will remember this moment, and do have a nice life."

SEXTET OF CLIENTS 161

Diplomacy coupled with honesty, the perfect combination in a trusted advisor.

KENNEDY CENTER HONOREE

For decades I have been the go-to person when it comes to choral conducting. I have spent my life successfully training choruses, including my own Robert Shaw Chorale. I even prepared the *Beethoven 9* chorus in 1945 for the historic Toscanini NBC Orchestra broadcast to commemorate the end of the war with Japan. What an honor when Toscanini himself called me the finest choral conductor he had ever worked with.

But that was thirty-five years ago, and now I want to be known as a conductor in my own right.

ML has come highly recommended and, when I meet with her, she asks one question: "What is it that you want to achieve if we work together?"

I reply that I want to be known as a great conductor.

She is very direct in her response and kindly says: "I can't do that. What I can do is to help position you as the greatest choral/ orchestral conductor in the world."

Her message is clear and deep in my heart, I know she is right. Go with strength and be the best in a specific niche—this really resonates. And so, I say, "Okay, we'll do it your way."

Ten years later, when I receive a 1991 Kennedy Center Honor, ML phones to say, "Congratulations on your well-deserved honor."

I reply, "I haven't forgotten where this all started—thank you!"

THE DIVA NEXT DOOR

My beloved voice teacher used to refer to me as "Renée Fleming, Mother Earth with a steel core"—a fair description.

As a young, up-and-coming, opera singer, I am told about ML by several prominent people. Over a six-year period, I interview with her three times.

The first two times, she listens intently, and says I am not quite ready for public relations and would be wasting my money to hire her. She adds that while she will not take me on just then, she remains interested but will understand if I want to go elsewhere. My decision—wait. I want to work with her.

I guess three is the charm, and in 1995, she says, "Yes."

Everything she does on my behalf for the next fifteen years helps build my career. Whenever I question a decision, she gives a solid, no-nonsense answer, and I know she is right.

Her strategy is impeccable, and I embrace her characterization of me as "the diva next door." The result is everything I have ever hoped for career-wise, and maybe even more.

We amicably part ways in 2010 and remain friends. To this day, though we no longer work together, I still call ML from time to time on sensitive issues, and she is always there for me.

JUILLIARD PRESIDENT

ML and I, having been friends now for more than a decade, frequently have philosophical discussions about what young artists need to know and are not being taught in conservatories.

As we return to New York City from judging a 1995 national music competition in Michigan, we are chatting yet again about this topic in an airport lounge. Spontaneously, I tell her that I want her to join the faculty at Juilliard.

She laughs and says: "Joseph Polisi, are you serious? To teach what?"

I ask if she would like to create a course about reality, specifically for singers, filling the void we have been talking about for years. If not now, when?

She loves the idea and welcomes the challenge of developing a syllabus that would cover all aspects of real life for musicians. Privately she calls it "Reality 101."

She has two requests: First, that the course—available to fourth-year undergrads and first-year graduate students—be mandatory for graduation, and second, that she be free to present opinions that may occasionally be contrary to school policy. I agree to both.

The results over the next twenty-two years prove invaluable to the young singers. They cannot get enough of her "real life" advice—some even take the class a second time.

Our dean summed up her tenure at Juilliard when he told her: "If you are ever having a bad day, just come by my office and read the comments on file from your students. They adore you and are so grateful for the enormous amount of practical and real information you have shared."

ML AT LA SCALA

Well, I have made it to La Scala, formally known as Teatro alla Scala.

You can imagine how excited I am, being of Italian descent, to be hired to promote a major US tour for the most celebrated opera house in Europe, or maybe the world.

Little did I know that this honor would come with a Faustian bargain.

Visiting *bella Italia* has always been pure heaven. With friends in both the north and the south of Italy, it has been a favorite and frequent place to vacation. Working there turns out to be quite another story.

I am far from fluent in Italian, as my parents used it at home when they didn't want us to understand what was being said. But even with my limited ability, Italians are encouraging, and I can make myself understood.

In the early 1990s, when Riccardo Muti suggests that I handle public relations for the La Scala tour of the United States, I am elated. He is currently La Scala's music director and, having worked with him in other organizations over many years, I know we are simpatico.

I am nervous and excited as I prepare for my first meeting in Milan. I am taking private conversational Italian lessons and even write the contract for La Scala in Italian, just to be safe.

Off to Italy I go, contract in hand, to see the top administrator, the *intendant* of the opera house. After chatting with him in Italian and English, I say: "Well, I think we agree on all the terms, so here is the contract reflecting everything we have just discussed. Shall we both sign it?"

He smiles most charmingly and says, "*Signora*, we are both Italians, so there is no need for a contract."

I answer, "*Dottore*, that's exactly why we need one!" We both sign, but little did I realize how worthless it would be.

The project ebbed more than it flowed over the next few years. When the Italian government is involved, change is inevitable. What started as a major US tour, with multiple productions in several major cities, is ultimately reduced to two performances of the Verdi *Requiem* with the La Scala Chorus and Orchestra at New York's Carnegie Hall—albeit two glorious concerts in the hands of the legendary Maestro Muti.

During this three-year project, which included several trips to Milan, I designed, discarded, redesigned, and finally executed a public relations plan for the La Scala visit. Expenses were mounting and nothing had been paid, not even a portion of my fee. It is now one week before the entire company is to arrive in New York City.

I phone La Scala and get through to the *intendant*, a miracle in itself, and calmly state, "*Dottore*, you know I have worked on your project for three years now. I am sure you are aware that La Scala owes me a great deal of money."

He replies, "*Cara Signora, non è un problema*. Don't worry, you will be paid after our New York trip."

Seeing nothing but red flags, I quickly say, "Please understand that this is a serious matter. If the entire amount you owe is not wired into my bank account within forty-eight hours, there will be a work stoppage and nobody in New York, or for that matter in the United States, will know that you and your company are here." A total bluff on my part to be sure, but the *intendant* has no idea, as a work stoppage is always possible in Italy.

As it turns out, the entire princely sum is wired into my account within twenty-four hours, well ahead of the deadline. All goes as planned with excellent coverage. Everyone is happy. And as for the *intendant*, he never suspected that I was bluffing.

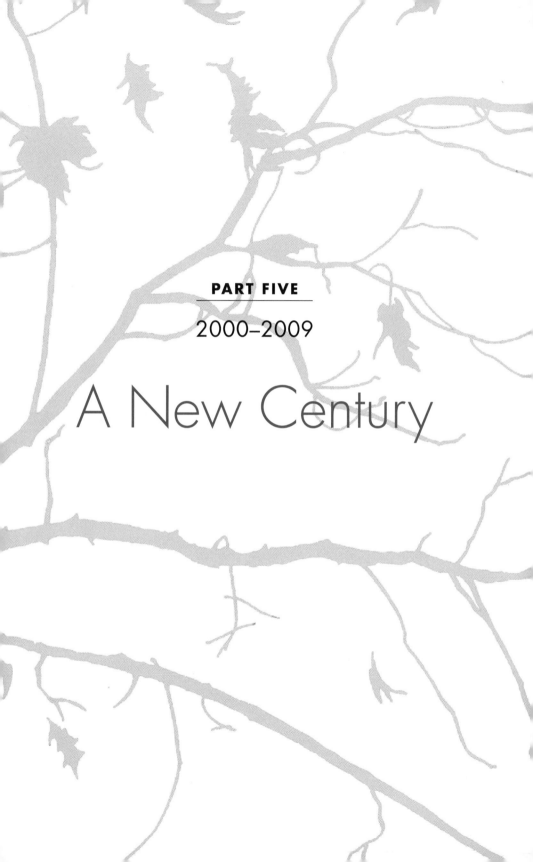

PART FIVE

2000–2009

A New Century

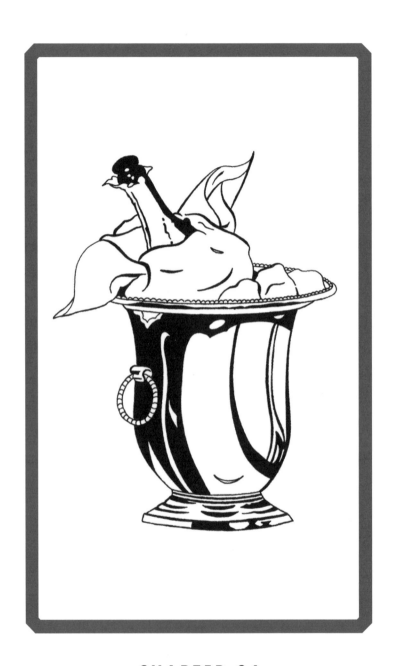

CHAPTER 36

NZ and the Millennium

ADVENTURES ABOUND, AND TRAVELING WITH SOME-
one who enjoys exploring as much as I do is a complete
joy. Together Nicky and I had many opportunities to experience the world—sometimes for business, other times for
sheer pleasure, and oftentimes for both. We tended to have
unusual and non-touristy experiences, in large part thanks
to Nicky's friendly and thoughtful ways of appreciating
the people we encountered. He made friends everywhere.
Each year, no matter where else we might travel, we would
make it a point to visit our favorite spots: Ogunquit, Maine,
and Paris, France. What a joy to walk into our favorite
Maine emporium, Amore Breakfast, and be greeted by the
proprietress with a big hug and cups of coffee, or to go
into Muscade, a Paris bistro, and have the proprietor race
to the front door shouting "Nicky!" and immediately bring
two glasses of champagne to toast our return. We enjoyed
marking special occasions, like the millennium, with close
Parisian friends.

Where have the decades gone? Ever since my 1950s rock 'n'
roll days, I've loved sharing that wild, almost surreal era
with my friends. So, why should the millennium be any different?

ML and I decide to celebrate the turn of the century in Paris with our close French friends. The night is magical. I am in my element playing keyboard and singing rock 'n' roll hits from the fifties and sixties (my own included), while regaling everyone with stories from those halcyon days. My other passion that night is dancing with my love, ML: We jitterbug to Jerry Lee and slow dance into the wee hours to Sinatra and Aznavour, our backdrop the twinkling light show of the Eiffel Tower. What a glorious time to be alive—to be alive and in Paris!

Come to think of it, our most special New Year's Eves have all been in France. In the early 1990s, we are invited to Tulette, where another French family is in the process of renovating an old stone house in the middle of a vineyard. ML, who makes all our social arrangements, gets the message wrong, unusual for her. But they are speaking quickly in French, and as she says, "My French is barely passable and nothing more." She mistakenly thinks our friends are saying they have finished their renovation, when actually they are just at the beginning. She does get the part right about being sure to wear very warm and old clothes. When we arrive for New Year's Eve, we find out why the dress code is so important.

The house, standing in the middle of nowhere, is just a shell—four walls, a roof, barely running water, a stove, a few space heaters, and no front door, just a big blanket that is no match for the raging mistral winds whipping through the vineyards. A dining table and six chairs complete the indoor picture. Calling the setting rustic would be an exaggeration.

We are given a choice—we can dine, or we can be warm, but not both. We choose the oven and our hostess's spectacular delicacies over the space heaters. You see, using both at the same time would blow out what little power there is.

So, keeping on layers and layers of warm clothing, we eat like kings and between courses warm our fannies in front of a huge roaring fire. Of course, the red wine and champagne are in never-ending supply, adding to our warmth.

Years later, to ring in 2001, we return to the same setting, now fully renovated and beautiful, and, oh, yes, this time with plenty of heat as well as food. It's a house party for twelve, including the original six from years back. Since ML and I have come the farthest, we are given the master guest room and retire around 2:00 a.m., well before everyone else. A few hours later, we are awakened by a commotion in the living room. Curiosity gets the better of us, and we throw on our clothes to rejoin the festivities. Of course, it's no secret that I can always be tempted by red wine, but drugs have never held any appeal, not even at the height of my rock 'n' roll days. Greeted by a sea of white faces, I quip, "No one told us about the Pillsbury bakeoff," which sends the already raucous room into gales of laughter, and the party rocks until dawn. Happy is the new year, the new decade, the new millennium! *Salut!*

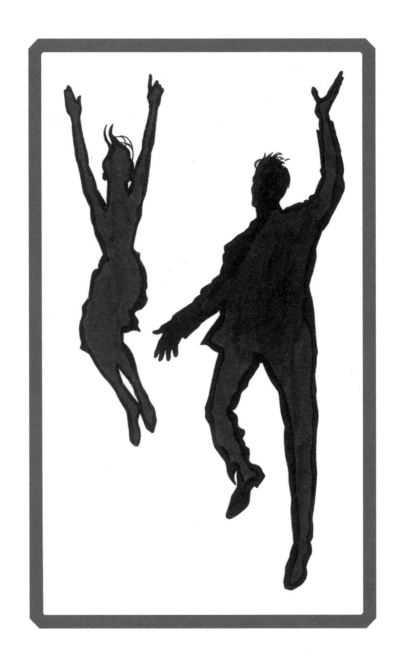

CHAPTER 37

NZ, Full of Surprises!

NICKY NEVER LIKED SURPRISES, WHETHER IT WAS A gift or an event. I, on the other hand, have always loved to be surprised. And surprise me he would, like bringing a weekly rose (a throwback to earlier days) or spontaneously putting on a Sinatra CD so we could slow dance in our living room. When I turned sixty, Nicky outdid himself in the "almost surprise" department, soon to be revealed. When I reached my seventieth birthday, he asked if I wanted a repeat of my sixtieth. I opted instead for a trip to Sicily with dear friends, wanting to walk the streets of Noto where my Falcone grandparents had walked more than a century before. He was happy to oblige, and the Sicily trip turned out to be the most wonderful gift—fulfilling, sentimental, and energizing for all of us. Nicky's ever-present thoughtfulness showed in all that he did.

ML is turning sixty—it seems impossible, but it's true. A few of her friends have reached out to me about throwing her a surprise party. Great idea, but their ideas about what to do and mine are not in sync.

I agonize. While I want to surprise her, I need her guidance to corral her friends and make sure this party comes off perfectly. If

I tell her, no one must ever know. For weeks, more agony until I finally decide to tell her and, while I'm sure she would have preferred to be surprised, she knows me so well and appreciates that this is the way I have to do it.

I invite a hundred of her nearest and dearest, and yes, they all show up, even her ninety-year-old mother, Gammy, who is front and center to greet her as she enters the restaurant to the roar of "Surprise!" ML plays her part to the hilt. What a special moment. The surprise is complete, and no one is any the wiser.

I am so proud of this celebration. My loving caricature of her as the symbol of the evening graces everything: the invitation, the cover of the remembrance book, and the party favors—a coffee mug and the bottle of fragrance created for the occasion by a friend who is considered one of the great "noses" in the perfume business. A cousin, who just happens to be a professional baker, has created a cake to look like the pleats of the Issey Miyake dresses ML favors, and the Italian food and wine flow all evening. Instead of indulging in a bunch of talking head tributes, always a bore especially when everyone wants to speak and many don't know when to stop talking, we present her with a special leather-bound book of written remembrances, the kind you dream of and usually get only at your funeral.

She is sooooo happy, and that makes me sooooo happy. I am basking in compliments from everyone about how flawlessly I have pulled off the event and, of course, I share the credit with her friends. As I catch the eye of my secret, silent partner, she gives me the biggest wink.

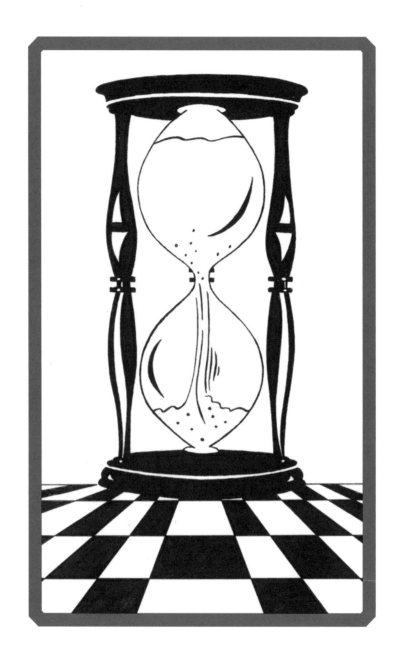

CHAPTER 38

Gammy's Caregiver

THERE HAS TO BE A SPECIAL PLACE IN HEAVEN FOR professional caregivers. They are extraordinary people, devoting their lives to helping others live to the fullest, especially toward life's end. In our family, our own personal guardian angel who looked after my mother was Georgian-born Silva Khundiashvili. In Georgia (once part of the Russian Empire and later of the Soviet Union), Silva had been a banker; in the United States she cared for others while subsidizing her whole extended family back home.

I have always called Silva my sister and made sure that at my mother's funeral she sat in the family pew with my brother, sister, and me. Silva was like a loving daughter to Gammy, my mother, always understanding how difficult it was for this proud and fiercely independent woman to accept help—help that Silva gave with great kindness, never treading on Gammy's dignity.

ML's mother, Mary, is called *Gammy* by her whole family. I meet Gammy on her ninetieth birthday. Her children throw her a big restaurant party, inviting relatives and friends. It is a beautiful celebration, and I am there as a caregiver for one of her friends, a neighbor of almost fifty-five years. Gammy's family makes me feel welcome, and I can see they are good people—loving, warm, and caring. Two years later, when their lovely neighbor passes, Gammy's family sees a perfect opportunity to get some much-needed help. But Gammy is still strong and independent and wants to do everything herself, just as she has for ninety-two years. To give you an idea, the family recently put its collective foot down because Gammy was seen hanging out of a second-story window cleaning the outside glass—she is one of a kind. Her family knows Gammy needs a twenty-four-hour, live-in person to ensure her safety. The decision can't be put off much longer.

When ML hires me on behalf of the family, my move is overnight—from one end of the street to the other. The siblings appreciate my work and often tell me so. They understand how challenging and difficult caregiving can be, not only for me but for their strong-willed mother.

Gammy adores her three children along with ML's partner, NZ—she calls him her fourth child. Her daughter Angel lives nearby, her son, Louis, lives in Los Angeles, and ML lives in New York City with NZ. Everybody is involved in taking care of Gammy. Angel visits often, ML and NZ come out to New Jersey almost every weekend to see her and give me some time off, and Louis calls often and visits when he can. They all check in daily, at least by phone.

Gammy's family adores and appreciates her and how hard she has worked all her life. They agree, now is her time to rest and enjoy life without worry, and of course, be safe, which is easier said than done.

I spend two years caring for Gammy and the home she loves and has fought hard to keep—it is where she is happiest. Her children promise that they will never move her out, a promise they keep.

During Gammy's last days, ML, sitting by her bed, gently says, "If you want to let go, it's okay because our family is together, and we will stay close. And I will still talk to you every morning as I always have."

Gammy, who has been sleeping most of the time, makes a very quiet, hard-to-hear comment.

Shocked, ML looks at NZ saying, "Did she say what I think she said?"

He nods yes.

What Gammy has said in her typical, slightly teasing way is, "Who cares." It makes us all laugh.

On a very cold Sunday about a week before she dies, her loved ones gather by her side. Gammy asks to see each of us separately, me included, saying, "Silva, you are my family too."

Later we share what she has said to each of us: "Thank you for taking such good care of me."

Her beautiful spirit passed on January 12, 2009, exactly one month after her ninety-fourth birthday, and her once-bustling house, the center of her life for many happy years, fell silent.

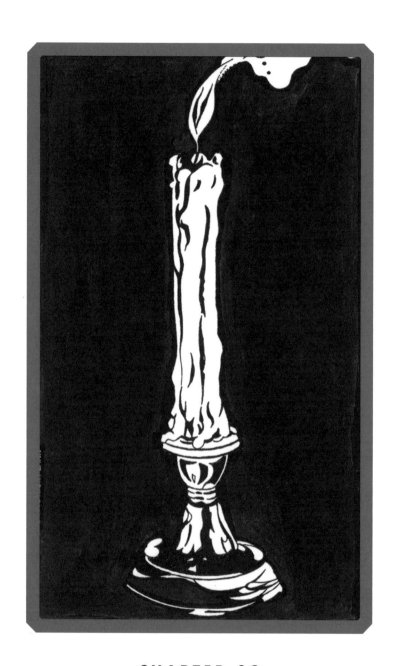

CHAPTER 39

Reflections on Gammy

MY STRONGEST EMOTIONS ARE MORE CLEARLY shared in poetry. While I don't write with any regularity, life-changing events often compel me to use the brevity and succinctness of poetry to share my deepest thoughts.

THE THANK-YOU

One day and one week to go,
Realization that death is imminent.
Coming out of a long reverie, she summons her loved ones.
To each, she whispers a thank-you of goodbye,
Hands held tightly, eyes locked in love for one last
    penetrating time.
Those eyes, having seen nine plus decades, close,
To dream again
Closer to the light.
A week and a day pass . . . silence.

THE CLOSING

She leaves her home for the last time,
Carried to eternity.
The emptiness is immediate.
Without her presence the space becomes just a house
Waiting to be a home again.

MY GAMMY

Heart, smile—Her essence.
Strength, determination—Her life.
Dignity, grace—Her legacy.
Calm . . .
Final peace.

LONELINESS

The loneliest time is forgetting and going for the phone,
Then remembering that the line is dead.
The voice of memory echoes, "Who cares"—
A line that still brings a smile, remembering the day when
    resignation sighed these sentiments,
Half in jest, half in truth.
"I will talk to you every morning, just as I always have in life."
The quiet, almost inaudible response, "Who cares."
Not wanting to trust the sounds,
I check with my soulmate sitting on the other side of the bed.
"Yes, you heard correctly," comes the bemused answer.
The memory of "Who cares" still evokes a smile.
How direct, how playful, how real, how resigned . . .
How Gammy.

FIRST ANNIVERSARY

An eternity or the blink of an eye.

Time passes,

With each moment a precious reminder of what really
matters.

Thoughts of those last moments linger—

Peace,

No longer needing the brave, heroic heart to beat.

The soul remains, hovers

Before moving on.

Visitations,

A gentle reminder of the gifts left behind,

Never forget to LOVE.

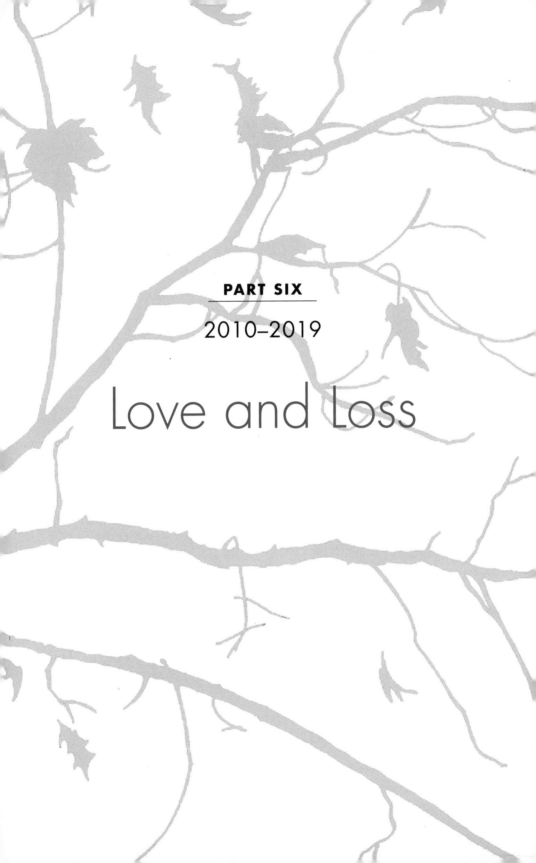

PART SIX

2010–2019

Love and Loss

CHAPTER 40

Marriage, Valentine's Day, a New Heart

Marriage is a wonderful institution, but it's not for everyone. For years my mantra was: "We are together because we choose to be. Why potentially spoil it with a piece of paper?" That's precisely why I said "no" to Nicky's many proposals of marriage over a thirty-year period . . . and then, one fateful day, I needed to pop the marriage question myself, and it was Nicky who said "*yes*!"

This is a love story, focusing on three days in February, a grand trifecta destined to change the course of our beautiful lives forever.

By this time, Nicky and I have been together for thirty-four years and, periodically, he asks me to marry him.

My answer is always the same, "Why change what is perfect?"

And so, in early February of 2017, it totally surprises him when I, seemingly out of the blue, say, "Why don't we get married?"

To which he replies, "Why, after all these years, this sudden change of heart?"

My answer to him: "We clearly are still very much in love; we are in our seventies and not getting any younger. Why not?"

But the truth is—I am very worried about him and have been for many months. What specifically prompted my marriage proposal? During a recent cardiologist's visit, an appointment was quickly made to do an angiogram on Valentine's Day. "Doesn't everyone check their heart on this day?" was my quip, just to make a heavy situation a bit lighter.

And so, on February 13, after decades of everyone assuming we are married, we say our vows at City Hall, and become husband and wife. It's simply a legality, but also a blessing, given what's to come.

The next day we "newlyweds" spend Valentine's Day at the hospital, hoping that the scheduled angiogram is just a routine precaution, the worst outcome perhaps being a stent. What is clear, as we sit together in the hospital waiting room holding hands, is that we have never been more in love.

My concerns turn out to be justified—oh, how I would have loved to be wrong! The angiogram results are shocking. It's the worst news possible: All four arteries are clogged, blocked at 100 percent, 99 percent, 80 percent and 50 percent. How Nicky was still running up and down subway steps that very morning is a complete mystery. The doctors tell us to go home and schedule an appointment for surgery. Completely shocked by the news and even more shocked at the suggestion of going home, I quickly compose myself and calmly say: "I don't think so. We are not going anywhere. You have just given us disastrous news, so I think we will stay right here until your top surgeon is summoned to review this report."

The triple bypass surgery is scheduled for the next morning.

How ironic that Nicky, the man with the biggest heart in the world, turns out to be the one with heart problems.

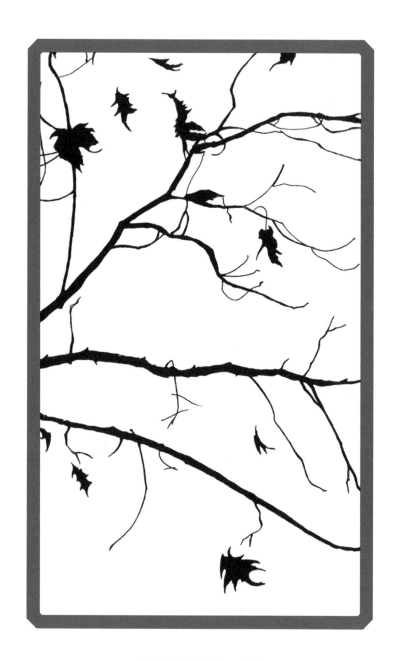

CHAPTER 41

NZ Asks, "What's Happening to Me?"

I am so happy to be here to tell the tale. Never did I dream that my heart would be a problem.

For months I was feeling so tired, foggy, and occasionally confused. While ML and I are in Vienna to usher in 2017, odd things are happening. I black out on New Year's Eve in the hotel lobby and pretend to have tripped as I quickly come to. Then there's the night between Christmas and New Year's Day when I get lost walking to meet ML and friends at a nearby restaurant I know well. I am angry at ML for not writing down the address, and I've left my cell phone in New York so I can't call her. After an hour of aimlessly wandering and still not finding the place, instead of panicking, I just stand very still near St. Stephen's Cathedral, hoping ML will get my vibe and come looking for me. A similar miracle happened once twenty-five years earlier in Japan, when we magically found each other walking down a secluded street. So, maybe it can happen again. I can only imagine how worried she must be. She does come looking for me, and we're reunited. Lucky again. As we join our friends, now an hour and a half late, which is so unlike me, my embarrassment subsides as they are visibly relieved that I am all right.

From Vienna we travel on to Paris, where one night I awake drenched in sweat, shivering, and suffering from major indigestion. By morning, I am fine and think nothing of it.

Later in January 2017, I am in my doctor's office for my usual six-month physical and happen to ask about the results of a test I had taken six months earlier—a calcium score test. When I look at the doctor's face turning white as a sheet, I know trouble is brewing. The score is seriously off the charts, dangerously high, and he neglected to flag it when he should have. Now wasting no time, he gets me to a top cardiologist.

The cardiologist, whom I immediately trust and like, gives me the bad news following an angiogram: I need serious surgery, triple bypass surgery. This is the last thing ML and I expected to hear.

Surgery the next day is intense and long. I am following the bright, comforting, white light, but suddenly I stop my peaceful departure. No, I can't do this. I can't leave ML now—after all, we've been married only two days! I need to come back to her for just a bit longer.

The hospital recovery period is brutal, complete with wild, horrible hallucinations. I can't get a grip. Everyone chalks it up to the anesthesia, but honestly, the hallucinations and fogginess never completely subside in the months that follow. One very mean nurse thinks there is a major problem brewing, but because she's so abrasive, no one pays much attention to her warnings. I can't wait to be home with my "new" wife, where I know I will be safe. The heart is now fixed, but the aftermath doesn't bring any clarity of thought or renewed energy either. I keep thinking this will just take more time. Yet, I can't help wondering, "What's happening to me?"

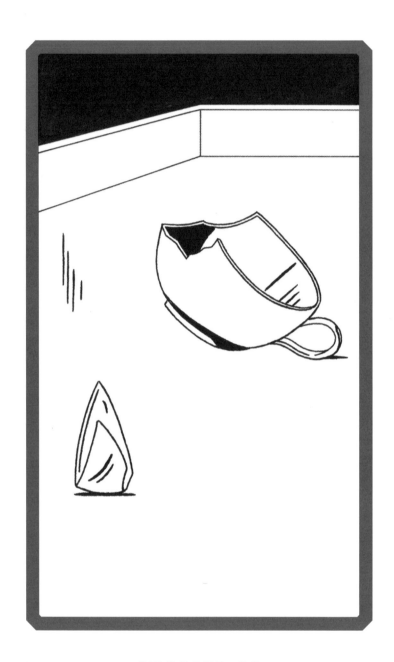

CHAPTER 42

Lifelong Friend MB Remembers

MARY BETH PEIL (MB) IS KNOWN AS AN ACTOR'S actor, always in demand. The fact that she was available to come to Stockholm with Nicky and me was nothing short of a miracle. When I asked her to host the Birgit Nilsson centennial event at least a year in advance of the 2018 celebration, little did I know what a major turning point this trip would turn out to be or how much I would really need her there as a friend. From the moment MB, Nicky, and I entered John F. Kennedy International Airport bound for Stockholm, I knew what I had been fearing for a while was real—Nicky's recently repaired heart was not the reason for many of the unusual things happening to him. I had pushed the envelope to the limit with this trip, and it was clear that something else was desperately wrong with my beloved husband. I needed to get on it, to find the reason and then the solution. Lights, camera, action!

Until now, I have never heard ML utter the words, "MB, this might have been a bad idea." For years, ML and NZ have loved traveling together. Hearing her say this, I am very glad I am traveling with them, so I can help.

When she invites me to come to Stockholm to be the mistress of ceremonies at the centennial celebration for the legendary Swedish soprano Birgit Nilsson, I am beyond delighted. Then to discover that my schedule is clear for the month of October 2018, well, I know this is meant to be—my answer, a resounding "yes."

As we three arrive at JFK Airport, I notice that NZ is in a complete fog, unable to navigate the long lines by himself. I also notice that my dear friend ML is doing everything for him, almost leading him by the hand under the guise of loving gestures.

We make it to Stockholm, where it becomes clear that NZ is not up to this trip. ML knows it too, but here we are. She is pretty much in charge of the whole elaborate Stockholm event and is there to work, day and night. NZ is an invited guest, so his presence is requested only at official evening events.

God bless NZ. He immediately recognizes that he is very low on energy and must find a way to be there for ML when it counts. So, they arrange a routine. He joins her for a large breakfast each morning in the hotel dining room, and she accompanies him back to their room, as he is having a bit of trouble finding it by himself. He sleeps all day as she works. She comes back to him in the late afternoon in time to help him dress for the evening's festivities. Once they arrive at the scheduled event, it's like he turns on the switch and is his charming, witty, and interesting self. The toll it takes on him is enormous. This goes on for three days and three nights, and he knows exactly how to conserve the energy that he needs to make it through.

On one free evening, a few of us go out for a low-key dinner, and NZ is looking forward to being with us. On the walk to the restaurant, I walk with him arm in arm and suddenly I feel him falling to the ground, taking me with him. I know from ML that this also happened earlier in the month in New York. It's very concerning.

I observe how lovingly they work together, as they always have. He knows that he is not up to the tasks at hand, and yet seems to want so badly to be there for her. It takes every ounce of his strength to attend the requested events and then to be his entertaining self in a crowd.

She has the routine down and despite the enormous business responsibilities on her shoulders, she is always there for him. Their teamwork is truly stunning.

I am so happy to be there in my official capacity, but even more, I am happy to be there as a friend to them both.

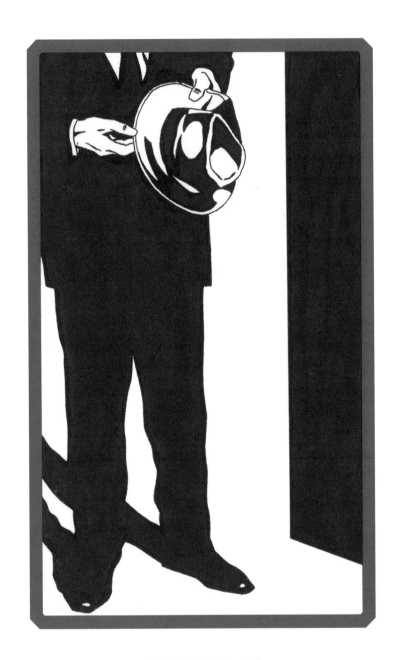

CHAPTER 43

When Nicky Met "Lewy"

nitially it was a relief to believe that Nicky's heart was the culprit. Having experienced from him a bit of erratic behavior, forgetfulness, fatigue, occasional anger, and paranoia during 2016 into 2017, finding out that he needed triple bypass surgery came as a welcome solution, or so we thought.

The long, involved surgery of February 2017 was pronounced a success. All arteries were repaired, but a lot of anesthesia was involved, with the aftermath being severe hallucinations. We were assured that this always happens with open-heart surgery and there was nothing to be alarmed about. The head nurse, brutal and autocratic, was not so sure. She was signaling that more might be going on in the brain, but because her bedside manner was so obnoxious, what she was implying was dismissed. That is, until much later.

When Nicky was finally released from the hospital, he was relieved to be home. During his ten-day ordeal, he had lost ten pounds from his already slight frame, and we faithfully followed all instructions to help him regain his weight, plus strength and acuity. But none of this happened.

Over the next six months, instead of gaining weight, Nicky lost even more, which was alarming, to say the least. He had no energy and would have to nap a great deal. And, worst of all, he seemed to be forgetting things . . . nothing too serious, but enough for me to start keeping a notebook.

My monitoring and note taking extended for another twelve months, all the while hoping and praying for improvement. There was none. Having changed our primary-care physician in June 2018, I was concerned enough by late November of that year, just after our alarming trip to Stockholm, to ask our new doctor for a baseline MRI.

What I had been witnessing, but keeping to myself for months, were occasional hand tremors while Nicky was awake and asleep; talking in his sleep while experiencing dreams that seemed real; shuffling while walking but able to correct it when reminded; speaking haltingly and searching for words (this from a guy who was quick with words and a great storyteller); having short-term memory lapses (he usually remembered everything); leaving the water running in the bathroom or kitchen; occasionally leaving the gas on and kitchen cabinet doors open; becoming very dependent; feeling uncomfortable going to appointments alone; experiencing high anxiety; speaking erratically so it was harder than usual to follow his conversation; and he had been working on the same painting for almost two years, which was not his work style.

Nicky himself began to be alarmed about his weight loss despite eating well, and noticed he was dreaming about falling. He was beginning to be aware of mental changes, not the least of which was thinking his dream activity was real. And it would take him twenty minutes to write one check. Something was definitely wrong.

The MRI of January 2019 showed no big surprises: for a seventy-five-year-old man, his brain looked age-appropriate. There had been no strokes or mini-strokes, but there was microvascular disease with the arteries of the brain closing a bit, similar to what happens in heart disease. We were told that this could be helped with a good diet, exercise, and control of cholesterol and diabetes. By late January, however, our physician was concerned enough, prompted by my continued description of cognitive problems and short-term memory loss, to send us to a first-rate neurologist to see if Parkinson's disease and dementia could be ruled out.

During our first neurology visit, mid-February 2019, extensive cognitive testing was done, and the neurologist clearly stated that Nicky had Lewy body dementia with Parkinsonian aspects, a progressive disease with no cure. This was based on testing along with Nicky's description of cognitive difficulties and physical problems including falls, fatigue, and hallucinations—mostly hearing voices.

What followed was a DaTscan procedure and a REM sleep test, both used in Nicky's case as additional tools to support an LBD diagnosis. At a follow-up visit on March 1, 2019, Nicky learned that the test results did indeed support the Lewy body dementia diagnosis. Little did we know at the time how unusual it is to get an LBD diagnosis on the first try!

As background, here's what the Lewy body dementia diagnostic criteria can include: progressive cognitive decline; fluctuations in alertness; lack of clarity/fogginess interfering with ability to work, socialize, and multitask; sleepiness; visual and/or audio hallucinations; delusions; REM sleep behavior disorder, where dreams are physically acted out; depth perception issues; and more often than not Parkinsonian symptoms (for example tremors, balance issues, slowness of movement, rigidity of arms and legs). What one could expect from LBD with Parkinsonian aspects over time is the body eventually shutting down, with symptoms like a hoarse voice; swallowing issues; lack of strength in the hands; walking more slowly and eventually perhaps not being able to walk at all; major cognitive difficulties, and the list goes on. What makes it all the more difficult is that no two cases are alike.

For Nicky, the only medication prescribed by the neurologist was donepezil (the generic form of Aricept), which could possibly serve to boost any good areas of the brain. With LBD, new medications are introduced one at a time to see how they actually work. The key is to go low and slow—start with a low dose and slowly add more as needed.

All of this was a lot to process. I thought about all that had been revealed and made the decision to discuss almost everything with Nicky, for which he was grateful. Some of the more alarming aspects I chose to leave out. Together we decided that we would tell our family and friends clearly and simply what was going on. We wanted to avoid any discomfort or quizzical looks or speculation, and we encouraged them to be patient and to behave as normally as possible. We shared that Nicky might experience anger and anxiety that needed to be dealt with in the moment with kindness and clarity and patience.

Since the neurologist was brilliant at diagnosis (a blessing) but less forthcoming about what we could expect (a major disappointment), I was on my own. His only constructive words were that I would learn more from people experiencing LBD than I would from any other resource. Being annoyed and frustrated by his lack of answers to my questions, I combed the internet and went into a frenzy, actively seeking information and possible help. In the end, the neurologist was right. I did learn more from others going through similar experiences.

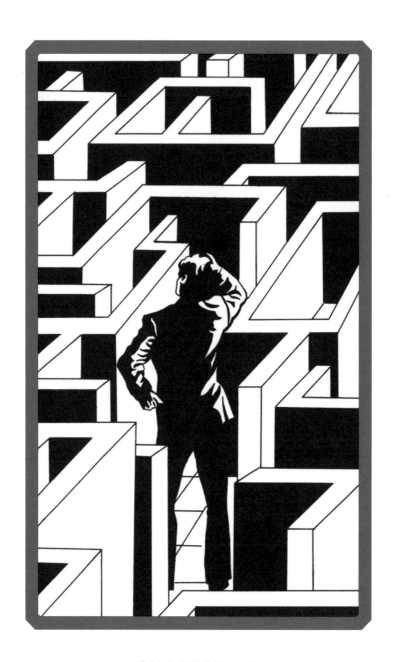

CHAPTER 44

NZ's New Doctor

NICKY CALLED OUR NEW PRIMARY CARE PHYSICIAN, John Cahill, "the angel," for indeed he was. Dr. Cahill's ability to see and act quickly gave us what most people dealing with LBD often do not get: the right path for a proper diagnosis on the first try—truly a miracle. I am sad to say that the norm is misdiagnosis, often multiple times, and sometimes never receiving a proper diagnosis at all.

Thank goodness for doctors who listen and respond. Nicky and I were fortunate to have had an excellent diagnostician for our first thirty years together, and it was a blessing to find a second excellent doctor in later life. It was not only the ability of Dr. Cahill to diagnose and treat that was so impressive, but also his humanity. He often seemed like a throwback to a more caring and gentler time when doctors really listened and weren't anxious to quickly usher you out of the office. This special physician walked the road with us, making a rough trek less frightening because he was compassionate and honest—both priceless attributes.

Even though I have known ML and NZ socially, they are new to me as patients. They come to me in June 2018, at a time when NZ is still recovering from triple bypass surgery. Even though it has been sixteen months since the surgery, he is not even close to being 100 percent, and this has been worrying them both.

During their October visit, ML asks if I would closely watch him, as she feels that his fogginess, fatigue, and confusion should have improved by now. She is very worried that something else might be going on, plus he has been unable to gain back the fifteen pounds he lost after the heart surgery. For someone who is slim to begin with, this is serious. She asks if we can do a baseline MRI of his brain. I tell her that I would like to monitor him a bit longer, that what she is seeing could be just age related.

She insists that it's something more, and I promise to keep an observant eye. By the end of the year, I conclude that she is right and schedule the MRI. It's now January 2019, and the MRI shows "age-appropriate deterioration."

Her answer is, "Fine, but what's next, because something is definitely wrong!"

As I watch, I have a pretty good idea of what it might be, having dealt with something similar in my own family. I send NZ to the best neurologist I know for testing. On March 1, 2019, the results are in, and the diagnosis is serious: Lewy body dementia (LBD) with Parkinsonian aspects. For this cruel disease, there is no cure and no slowing its debilitating pace. While it impairs cognitive ability and executive function, it also weakens motor skills. I truly hate that my hunch was correct.

I guess the moral here is to listen carefully to a tuned-in spouse. It is fortunate that ML kept insisting, and I heard her. For her and for me, there is some solace in giving a name to NZ's behavioral inconsistencies and symptoms, even though the prognosis is bleak.

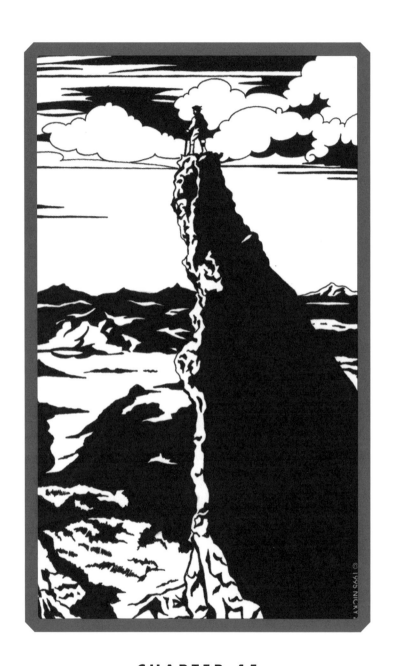

CHAPTER 45

NZ, the Fighter

hear the words *Lewy body dementia* loudly and clearly, and I know what they mean. Just minutes before, I had been joking with the neurologist as he pointed to a lion and asked, "What's this?"

My smart-ass answer: "Well. that's simple. That's my wife." My off-the-wall response slightly alarms him until ML quickly interjects that her birth sign is Leo—ah, now he gets the joke.

The neurologist says that to support the diagnosis, there are two more tests to be done—a REM sleep behavior disorder test and a DaTscan—but he is quite sure we are dealing with LBD. What I know instinctively is that I have received a death sentence. As my wife and I walk into the waiting room, I take her in my arms, look into her eyes and tell her that I have always wanted to meet her father, who died before we were together, and now, I am going to have my chance. She knows I understand exactly what is happening to me. I add, "My darling, we have had a great run together, we cannot be sad, but I will fight this with everything I have!"

The test results reinforce the worst—it is LBD. To be brave for my wife, the love of my life, and to bolster myself as well, I vow once again to fight it, to conquer it. I know full well that there is no stopping its progression, and she knows this too. I will die from it, that is certain. What is totally uncertain is the timetable of the disease—it could be a few years or longer. I am now in God's hands, and of course the expert hands of my primary care physician, John Cahill, whom I trust completely.

A few months later, when I am asked by the neurology team at NewYork-Presbyterian/Columbia Medical Center if I would address a group of forty interns on what I've been experiencing since being given the LBD diagnosis, I immediately say, "Yes," as it might help someone else. Mercifully, I am having a good day, and it's like being on stage during my rock 'n' roll days. I tell them candidly what LBD is doing to the quality of my life. I make them laugh, and I make them cry. The feeling in that moment is liberation!

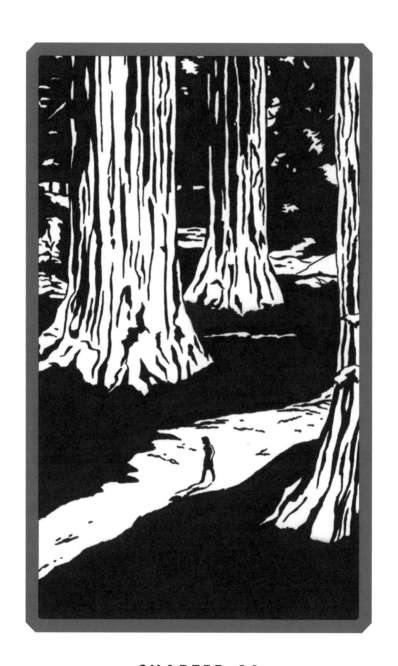

CHAPTER 46

"No, It Can't Be"

Upon hearing Nicky's diagnosis, my inner voice screams, *"Nooooo,* not my beautiful, brilliant husband."

And then the practical voice kicks in: "I need to find out more about this disease. I need to know what to expect. I need to know how to help him." Lewy body dementia is the most mysterious type of dementia, the one that draws blank stares from most people, even though 1.4 million people in the United States have been diagnosed with it. Knowing that LBD is the second most progressive form of dementia after Alzheimer's, I am counting on the neurologist for answers to my list of questions. To my surprise, he refuses to answer, no matter how many times I ask. I even ask Nicky to leave the room, thinking the doctor may not want to answer sensitive questions in his presence, but still nothing. I give up asking. I feel like an untethered balloon, left to float alone.

Turning my disappointment and then fury into action, I set about doing my own research. Thanks to a few friends, including the actor David Hyde Pierce, an organization devoted to helping families of those with dementia, CaringKind, is recommended to me. The people who run this organization give me general information about dementia in a warm, helpful, and friendly way, and offer many multitiered, free courses with titles like

"Understanding Dementia," "Family Caregiver Workshops," and "Legal and Financial Information." I sign up for and take them all, immersing myself in the world of dementia, hungry for any information they can provide.

Among the many wonderful things CaringKind provides is entrée to the Lewy Body Dementia Resource Center and its founder, Norma Loeb. When I phone the LBDRC helpline (833-LBD-LINE), Norma herself answers, and she along with her support groups, with their firsthand practical help, become my lifeline for the next two years. One of the first vital pieces of information Norma shares is that Nicky should carry an LBD Medical Alert Card (printed from the homepage of the Lewy Body Dementia Resource Center's website (www.lewybodyresourcecenter.org), because, should he ever be rushed to the ER, certain medications would be dangerous for him. Many medical professionals are not aware of LBD and could inadvertently cause serious problems with the wrong medications.

Basically from these two essential organizations, CaringKind and LBDRC, I learn that there are many types of dementia affecting approximately fifty-five million people worldwide—staggering numbers. The best known is Alzheimer's disease, and the least known is Lewy body dementia, with many others in between. Dementia is not a specific disease but rather is a general term for the impaired ability to remember, think, or make decisions, thus interfering with a person's daily life and activities.

Specifically about Lewy body dementia, I learn some startling facts:

- Lewy body dementia is the second most common form of progressive dementia after Alzheimer's disease and affects more than 1.4 million Americans. It is widely misdiagnosed, as it can mimic Alzheimer's disease, Parkinson's disease, or a psychiatric disorder.

- LBD is a neurodegenerative brain disease in which one size does not fit all, making it very hard to diagnose and, once diagnosed, difficult to treat and currently impossible to cure.
- More people have LBD than amyotrophic lateral sclerosis (ALS), muscular dystrophy, and cerebral palsy *combined*.
- More people have LBD than are HIV positive.
- Among those who have suffered from and lost the battle with LBD, in addition to my husband, Nicky Zann, are Tom Seaver, Dina Merrill, Estelle Getty, Casey Kasem, and Frank Corsaro. Through autopsy, it was discovered that Robin Williams also had LBD. And who knows how many others have been misdiagnosed?

At CaringKind, they share important tips about how to deal with people suffering from dementia in general: Show them patience and kindness and understanding, because a person with dementia cannot help his behavior, so it's up to caregivers to create coping mechanisms. Easy? No way. Important? You bet. It's the difference between helping someone maintain dignity or stripping them of it. And there are legal challenges too—for example, getting documents to protect the patient, primarily a last will and testament, health care proxy, and power of attorney.

At the Lewy Body Dementia Resource Center, I gain inspiration and solace from a like-minded set of caregivers, each facing some stage of the disease with a loved one. This group is made up primarily of women caring for their husbands or partners, occasionally an adult child who is caring for a parent, and more rarely a husband caring for a wife. The caregivers group meets twice a month to openly share experiences, letting other caregivers know they are never alone in this battle. The meetings are a lifeline and a blessing for which I am and always will be grateful. The group gets me through many extremely rough patches. There are also separate group meetings for those with the disease. The angel on earth, Norma Loeb, who founded and runs the organization, is a tireless advocate, consistently giving those in the group assistance and answers. Her kindness and expertise extend well beyond the groups to include the Resource Center's 365 days-a-year HELPLINE (833-LBD-LINE) and informative website (www.lewybodyresourcecenter.org). The tagline of LBDRC says it all—"bringing awareness, supporting with love."

Every caregiver dealing with LBD and other dementia is constantly reminded of a cardinal lesson: Caregivers must take care of themselves. The all-important question frequently asked: If something happens to you, who will be there to care for your loved one?

There are moments that are completely overwhelming, but we caregivers can never let this show. While our loved ones with LBD can't help or even always understand what's happening, they keenly sense emotions. Caregivers learn to develop their own survival tactics: deep breathing for calm, smelling lavender sachets, counting to ten before reacting, punching a pillow when no one is looking, and, a personal favorite, finding a private place to yell *fuck* at the top of your lungs. While this word is not part of my usual vocabulary, there is something about it that seems to alleviate pressure during those extremely stressful occasions. It's simply cathartic, and I share this with my fellow LBD caregivers, who at first find it amusing and then realize that it works. *Heck* or *darn* or *damn* just don't do it. It's important to do this all as privately as possible, trying never to let your loved one see your frustration, anger, or sadness . . . but do give yourself permission to be frustrated, angry, and sad! *It's okay.*

My thoughts these days often go back to my mother, the paragon of patience and my role model. For years from the mid-1950s onward, she was caring for the man she loved the most, too. Sometimes I think history is repeating itself, but then, so are the gifts of strength and courage.

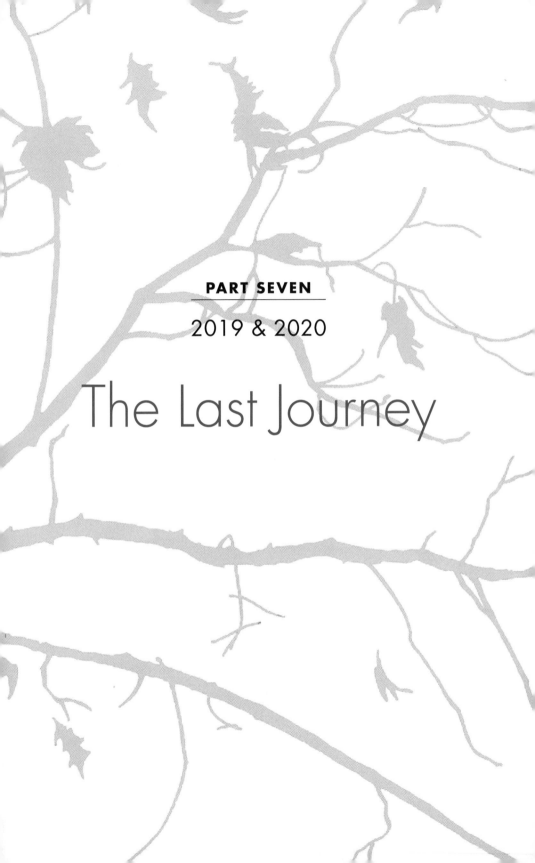

PART SEVEN

2019 & 2020

The Last Journey

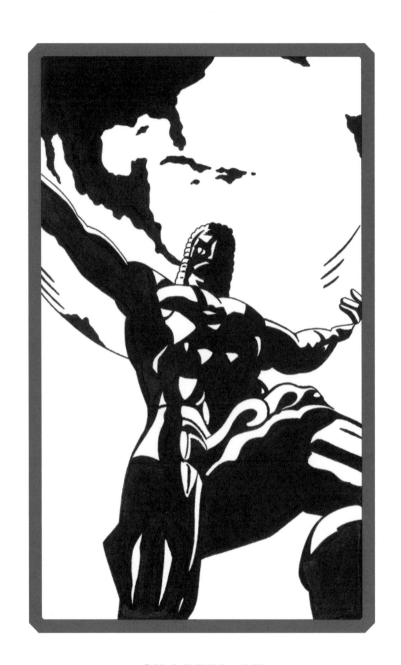

CHAPTER 47

Walking the Road Together

Our new reality is brutal—but hearing the LBD diagnosis does give my husband's condition a name (unlike Robin Williams, who never knew) and almost immediately provides a key to unlock an important door. Nicky now feels free to tell me about all the strange happenings that have been creeping into his daily life. For a while, he has been experiencing frequent auditory hallucinations. He hears voices coming out of the faucets and music coming out of the bedroom pillows. He asks if I hear them too. His legs begin to cramp and his back aches. Swallowing is difficult and hoarseness follows, and the weight loss continues to be seriously worrying. As time goes on, he fears incontinence, and his solution to combat that fear is not to eat. His constant fatigue makes any activity difficult, and his edginess occasionally leads to depression. He is obsessed with cleanliness and lives in fear of soiling himself. Even though he tries to mask it, I am aware of his fear and try not to show mine. These are the early days, and we are walking this unknown road together, still hand in hand.

A bit down the path, he begins to have nightmares, which, upon waking, turn into visual hallucinations—harmless creatures at first and then horrors. The norm becomes endless sleeping, which I don't disturb because I believe he needs it.

About four months into his illness, showering and dressing become more arduous. While he can still manage, it can take him up to two hours to complete these tasks. I just let him continue at his own pace. He shows occasional flashes of anger.

Summer comes, and we add speech and physical therapy to the regimen—both are working well, and he enjoys the stimulus. Socializing is still a treat and, being the consummate showman, he rises to every occasion, even though the payback is, you guessed it, more sleeping. I realize that one activity a day is enough for him, and this works reasonably well.

Now in August, we vacation in Maine at a resort we have been enjoying for thirty years. The change of venue triggers major disorientation, even though we book the same hotel room as before. The disorientation dissipates somewhat when we get a visit from our two-year-old godchild, Andrew, the apple of my husband's eye. To commemorate the visit, I am surprised and delighted when Nicky unexpectedly finishes a color pencil portrait of Andrew. It's a true miracle, because he hasn't been able to concentrate or draw anything for about a year. This is love speaking.

September 2019 marks the end of my beloved's independence. It's the moment I have been dreading and my heart breaks. A fall on the street when walking alone in our neighborhood signals that he now needs to be accompanied at all times. Despite his black eye, this new restriction does not sit well with him.

Hearing becomes an acute issue starting in October, plus he has greater difficulty distinguishing a dream from reality. His hands are visibly trembling—their strength gone—and his right foot is beginning to drag noticeably when he walks.

He rebels against his lack of independence, and in November he tests the water about going outside on his own. Determined, he tries it on a day when I am out at a meeting and immediately realizes it was a bad idea when, upon his return, he cannot get his keys to work in the door. Thank goodness for our wonderful doorman who helps him to get in. Mercifully, no harm done; this is the first and the last of such adventures.

Ah, the holidays are upon us. It's Thanksgiving and we are giving thanks in Maine at our get-away spot. This time it's a joyful and easy trip, but right on its heels comes more confusion in early December and a downward turn. For the first time I hear the words, "I am sick, I'm dying."

As we both cry in each other's arms, I add, "Sweetheart, we are all dying, just not today."

Despite his trouble standing up from a sitting position and the irreversible constant weight loss, we spend a wonderful Christmas with my brother, Louis, and sister, Angel. It's a love fest. Just after Christmas, as we start the new year 2020, godson Andrew, now almost three, accompanies us to the Christmas tree at Rockefeller Center. This proves to be the best tonic in the world for my dear husband, who is tired but happy.

In January and February, we visit MoMA and the Metropolitan Museum and the New York Philharmonic, big undertakings given his condition, but exhilarating too. We arrange as many lunches as we can with good friends, never more than four of us at a time, and these interactions are fun and stimulating, even though the next day Nicky is thoroughly exhausted.

He creates his last major work of art in February 2020. Determined to do a portrait in his signature style of India ink and magic markers, he brings godson Andrew's image to life in living color and presents it to him on his third birthday, February 15. This is a special bonding date for both Andrew and Nicky, because on that very day in 2017, Andrew was born at exactly the same moment as Nicky was being reborn through his heart surgery.

Studying the portrait, the birthday boy gleefully exclaims, "That's me," and runs to hug his godfather. It's a special moment—the artist at the finish line.

And then the world changes for all of us when COVID-19 strikes. Everything shuts down in New York City and isolation is mandatory starting in mid-March. While it's a devastating blow for most, for us it becomes a blessing. I can devote my full-time attention and activity to my husband's needs while keeping up with my daily work from home. Normally at this stage of LBD, we would be seriously looking to hire a caregiver, but this is COVID time, and bringing somebody into our home is simply not safe. I become his sole caregiver, and this turns out to be wonderful for us both.

Now I am able to be with him twenty-four hours a day. We cocoon. The Lewy body dementia goes in and out, as is its typical pattern, doing its dastardly best to keep him disoriented while keeping us both off-guard. A trademark of its cruelty is allowing him to be fully himself one minute, and then taking it all away the next. Each evening, no matter what, we sit down to dinner together in our dining room. Sometimes he eats, sometimes not; sometimes we talk, sometimes it's just silence. Then, under the guise of giving him a hug, I lift him gently as we then walk hand in hand to the bedroom and prepare for the remainder of the evening. Most nights, we are still holding hands as sleep descends.

COVID-19 confuses him, and it is an ongoing challenge to explain the restrictions and necessary precautions. Especially difficult for his affable personality is not being able to hug someone or shake hands, which he is constantly attempting to do when we are out for walks. Hand washing becomes a chore and sometimes a test of wills.

He has many more mood swings as he realizes he is declining. By the end of March, after one exhausting exchange, he draws a very simple sketch of the two of us with masks, with the message: "You're only trying to help me. I'm so sorry!" My heart breaks yet again, and my tears flow.

April and May bring skirmishes about always needing to be helped and anger at having very little independence. He is now sleeping fifteen to twenty hours a day, and sometimes loses his voice completely. We are both aware that the end is near.

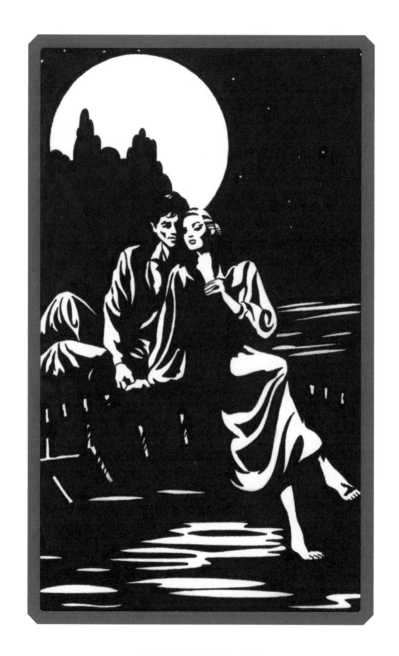

CHAPTER 48

NZ:
My Time Is Approaching

---

t's all right. You're dreaming, sweetheart." That has been your constant mantra, words that make me feel safe and calm.

I ask, "Did it happen?"

You say, "No it's the disease talking," a phrase that takes the sting out of my anger and fear. I feel confused, managed all the time.

You say, "You have every right to be feeling that way, because that's exactly what is happening."

I know you feel responsible for keeping me safe and out of harm's way.

The toll: You, Mary Lou, as wife, lover, and confidante, morph into my goddess of caregiving. Gone is the lover, replaced by pure love and so much responsibility.

My need for physical release seems to heighten as I lose control. I seek solace in a phone voice from the past, fulfilling my fantasy, keeping me calm and meaning nothing but release from tension. Bittersweet, it is a solution that restores my power in my otherwise powerless state. Mercifully, you understand and you don't judge. Sometimes when I can't dial the number, you do it for me.

Your goal is to uphold my most important wish—to keep my dignity intact while keeping me safe, and you do.

Your challenge: eternal patience and strength.

My challenge: to make sure I can still show you how much I love and appreciate you.

Our reward: loving smiles and constant hugs, both of us knowing deep inside that I trust you more than any human being on the planet.

I know your voice, your touch, your beautiful loving face—and then I don't. I am totally aware, and then oblivion. The last two months have been brutal. You, sweetheart, are the love of my life, my soulmate for eternity. I don't want to leave you, but this time, I know I must—my time is approaching. I am losing my strength. I weigh eighty-nine pounds. Even when I don't recognize you, I am somehow comforted by your presence, your gentle voice, your help in everything I do. Your loving hands are a sweet reminder of the past we have shared. There is a peace about leaving, a peace that even cuts through the fog in my brain. I decide in one of my more lucid moments to leave a poem for you, something that you will find after I am gone. When you do find it, hidden beyond some blank pages in the sketchbook next to my side of the bed, you will have no doubt that I knew all along what was happening. After the initial shock of discovery, I know it will give you comfort and strength.

Written in May 2020:

The photo on the wall
if I'm not mistaken, was
taken when our love was
just brand new
It was not long ago, when
we were making the plans,
to love each other strong
and be true
A devil in our home,
used deception to corrupt
the loyal angel that
my heart knew
An instant into this
cruel and hateful reception
vengeance replaced the heart that once
beat true
With blinding rage, and searing pain
a ready knife filled my hand
I thrashed with intent
cutting them down and never
was the same again
While I wait, for my date
with the hangman and his chore
and by chance I see my
reflection
that less than human sight that
haunts each tortured night
that stranger in the mirror is me . . .

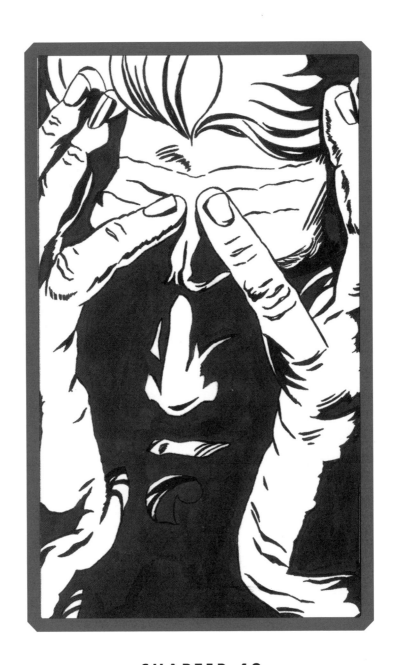

CHAPTER 49

Living with "Lewy":
LBD in Real Time

Through the entire experience with LBD, the Nicky I knew and loved never left but was sometimes held hostage by "Lewy," that unwelcome guest who would take over Nicky's identity for periods of time. When "Lewy" would appear, it was not my Nicky talking and acting out, it was the disease. This is something that I had to keep reminding myself.

One of Nicky's great and profound sayings was, "The pendulum swings; it just doesn't make any local stops." This can be applied to many things: history, current world events, relationships, social causes, and the list goes on. The only place this doesn't seem to apply is on the journey of life.

We are now about to make all the local stops on the LBD journey of the last two years of Nicky's life. This journey was to be the ultimate challenge and the ultimate act of love . . . helping the person I loved the most to exit this world with dignity and pride, and above all with love.

Starting with Nicky's official diagnosis of Lewy body dementia on March 1, 2019, I kept a monthly log of the fluctuations, so that all doctors involved could have the same monthly information on Nicky's condition. What follows is that log, punctuated by our emotional state and coping mechanisms. Our situation was further complicated by the severe isolation and restrictions imposed by COVID-19, which became both a blessing, as Nicky and I could be together twenty-four hours a day, and a curse, because the isolation did not allow for outside stimulation or help in caring for him.

This log vividly chronicles Nicky's actual decline and may be disturbing.

MARCH 2019

- Nicky tells me he has been hearing voices coming out of the faucet and music coming from the pillow. He asks if I too am hearing them. I tell him I don't hear what he is hearing, but I know that he is experiencing this and it's okay, I understand.
- His legs are cramping and achy (restless leg syndrome), and his back also begins to ache.
- There's a bit of trouble swallowing.
- Hoarseness creeps into his voice.
- At five feet, nine inches tall and normally weighing between 130 and 133 pounds, he is now at his lowest adult weight ever—106 pounds.

This first month is rough. I don't know where to turn. All I know is that I must learn everything that I can. I am like a madwoman searching for answers, searching for help, searching for some support. I feel so alone. The person that I would always turn to for advice, for solace, for help, for partnership, for love, my Nicky, was no longer able to provide most of these things. And yet, I needed to be sure to include him in everything that I could, so that he never felt left out or marginalized. We hugged each other a lot. We had always held hands, and now it seemed like I never wanted to let go of his hand. We tried to be as normal as possible . . . but what did normal mean now? I prayed a great deal, and I know Nicky did too. We went to St. Patrick's Cathedral and to the Church of St. Paul the Apostle to light candles with great frequency. We had our faith in God.

APRIL 2019

- Nicky's weight is down to between 104 and 106 pounds; he is resisting eating.
- The hoarseness in his voice continues.
- His skin is dry, more than usual.
- There is a bit of incontinence and a great fear of diarrhea.
- The audio hallucinations continue.
- There are some visual hallucinations.
- He has great fatigue.
- Edginess is creeping in, along with a bit of depression.
- He gets lightheaded.
- He is now obsessing over keeping himself clean and making sure he keeps the sheets clean; he is afraid of soiling himself and soiling the bed.

Realizing that his fear is heightening, being calm is a must. If there are any moments of soiling, I must keep those moments as light as possible. "It's no big deal," I tell him. "That's what washing machines are for." As for fatigue, I feel it's important not to push Nicky but to abide by what his body is saying.

He is always so upbeat, and to see him edgy and depressed breaks my heart. He keeps saying, "I am going to beat this," and my reply consistently is, "I know you are going to do the very best you can." I cannot bring myself to affirm his declaration of "beating this" as I know it's impossible. It's just too important, it's too painful, and I won't be cruel or undermining by verbalizing the brutal truth, but I also cannot bring myself to say, "Yes, you are right."

MAY 2019

- Nicky's weight hovers between 102 and 104 pounds.
- He references that he is not sure he can do the trip to Paris that we have planned for July; my answer, "Let's wait and see."
- Nicky and I are invited by the neurologist at NewYork-Presbyterian/Columbia Medical Center to give a lecture on May 21 for about forty interns and neurologists about what it feels like to be diagnosed with LBD. Nicky says yes to this, and he is a star! He is so happy to have been able to do this and to have succeeded. His sense of dignity is restored.
- He has a nightmare on May 26 about animals, especially squirrels, overtaking our bed. In the nightmare, he is also looking for holes in the wall to keep out mice. When he wakes from the nightmare around 2:00 a.m. and tells me about this, he is insistent that we buy a new $17,000 bed. Now fully awake in the middle of the night, he evidently sees a squirrel under me in bed (hallucination) and gets up and walks around the apartment to check the living room for more animals. He then goes back to sleep, and when morning comes and he is awake, he again sees a squirrel running around the bedroom and asks me about it. I assure him it is a hallucination. He is tired all day, has very loose bowels, has a slight accident, and claims not to be hungry—I am beginning to catch on that he is afraid to eat for fear of triggering diarrhea.
- Lots of fatigue is creeping in, with lots of sleeping day and night.

My heart is breaking. Paris is Nicky's favorite city in the world and for him to be backing away from going means that he is realizing how fragile he is. The bright spot of the month is watching Nicky speak to the doctors and interns at NewYork-Presbyterian/Columbia Medical Center. When we were asked to go there, I thought that I would be doing most of the speaking and that Nicky would participate in a public cognitive test. Boy, was I wrong. Nicky is having a particularly good day, he is feeling strong, he is feeling empowered. It's showtime! He takes the stage, and it is pure theater. He is the consummate performer as the showman comes to life making his audience laugh and cry and wildly applaud him and applaud his courage. I don't think I have ever been prouder of my Nicky or happier for him to have his dignity restored.

JUNE 2019

- Nicky's weight still fluctuates between 102 and 106 pounds.
- He has a bit of a queasy stomach along with discomfort.
- Periodic bouts of diarrhea continue with a few accidents.
- We add Glucerna nutritional drink to his daily diet, and this seems to help a bit.
- We now are careful to do just one activity a day (lunch or coffee or concert or dinner). Even one activity wipes Nicky out, and the next day he needs more rest.
- He is walking slower; a walk that used to take ten minutes, now takes at least twenty minutes.
- Daily grooming can take up to two hours, but I think it's important for him to exert his independence where he still can—showering, shaving, dressing.
- Great fatigue is still an issue.
- He talks in his sleep.
- He often thinks I am talking to him when I have not said a word.

- He is beginning to get a bit angry with me for my tone of voice and for not being responsive in the way he thinks I should be.
- My response: I am doing my very best to make him safe and comfortable, and I am truly sorry if there are times that I seem preoccupied and don't respond as he needs me to.
- Nicky has made the decision not to go to Paris. Travel is too stressful, and the fatigue level is too high. He and I are both afraid it would do more harm than good.

This is a huge turning point. When I mention to Nicky that if we go to Paris, we could facilitate our travel at the airports by ordering a wheelchair for him, his answer is an immediate and swift *"No wheelchair!"* And as he is refusing to use a wheelchair, his inner voice is telling him what he knows to be true—this trip is just too much. The sense of relief that comes when he makes that final decision is immediate, and I feel it is important for him to be the one to make that call.

JULY 2019

- July 3–4: Very social days with two late evenings of dinners with good friends; both visits, four hours each, are very positive and energizing.
- July 7: Nicky's weight is 102; he is angry and bored with any food, and he is trying to provoke arguments. There is general anger and acute fatigue.
- July 8: His weight is up to 103, and he is in a better mood.
- July 11: He begins talking several times a week to an old friend by phone, someone he hasn't spoken to in years. She seems to calm him down, and he can release tension when he speaks with her. She makes him happy; I suspect

the nature of the conversations is sexual, perhaps phone sex?

- July 13: He is looking more fragile.
- July 14: He weighs 102 and sleeps all day.
- July 15: It's early morning, and I notice Nicky is sleeping with his mouth distinctly skewed to the right. During his late morning nap, I notice the same thing. When he awakes, there is great fogginess, and he can't keep events of the day straight; he weighs an alarming 100.6 pounds.
- July 21: His weight is 100.3. He is extremely tired and sleeps most of the day.
- July 28: The weight is mercifully up to 103, but he is cranky about not exercising enough and feels dizzy, although that improves during the day.
- At the suggestion of the neurologist, he starts speech and physical therapy through Fox Rehab. They specialize in LBD, and their therapists are well trained; Nicky likes working in both areas and does well, especially in physical therapy, where he is immediately standing straighter, making him two inches taller.

The weight loss is frightening, and I try not to let my alarm show. Nicky's body is so fragile, and he is doing his very best to tone as much as he can with physical therapy. Appearance has always been important to him, and he makes the effort each and every day to be his tonsorial best. I admire this and his determination to make as much as possible work. He has remarkable will, but I need to be more quietly protective. I have realized that as much as he loves to be social, in addition to one activity a day, we now have to be cautious about planning two consecutive nights. It's just too much, and I have to monitor without seeming to take anything away.

AUGUST 2019

- August 1: There's a miracle: Nicky starts drawing a very beautiful portrait of our two-year-old godson Andrew. This is his first drawing in more than eight months, and it's a remarkable portrait drawn with India ink and colored pencils.

- August 2–4: There is great anxiety; the mornings are negative. Nicky needs sexual release, he feels guilty because of his July phone calls with his old friend, and then turns that guilt on me. My take, which I share with him: Nicky, you have to do what you need to do. On the positive side, he is eating well, sleeping well, and is generally sweet, very sweet.

- August 21: Nicky is sick with diarrhea and fatigue. I realize that we did too much the day before and Nicky can't handle it: a haircut, speech therapy, manicure and pedicure, drink at the end of the day with a friend. We need to slow down.

- August 26–September 1: We take a driving vacation to our favorite resort in Maine where we have been going for almost thirty years; Nicky is disoriented at night and sleeps fitfully with bad dreams. In the morning he wakes not knowing where he is, confused about the dreams and questioning if they are real. It takes two hours each morning to reacclimate, and then he is fine. The real bonus comes with a two-day visit from our two-year-old godson, Andrew, and his mother, Amanda, which brings Nicky great joy and energy.

This month the roller coaster is in full play. Emotions run high for Nicky, and his desire to do things is outweighed by the start of serious physical limitations. He wants to do what he used to do, but that is now impossible, and it's up to me to set the limits without making him feel the limitations are his fault. My new mantra is *there is no blame / there is no shame.* This is especially true in the arena of sex, which keeps coming into play. Each of us has just so much energy, and while I am blessed with an enormous amount of energy, there is a limit, and I know that my priorities are to be a loving wife, caregiver, friend, caregiver, companion, caregiver . . . you get the picture.

What I cannot continue to be is a lover. My love is as deep as ever, but my physical desire has turned a corner. I realize that Nicky still feels empowered in the area of sex: It seems to be something still within his control, and his need has been heightened. He has always been a sexual being, and now it might be the last vestige of his independence, of his manhood. While my energy just cannot go there, I recognize that since July, the telephone calls with the old friend—who lives hundreds of miles away and who has had an unreciprocated crush on Nicky for decades—have become more regular. I actually cannot remember how she resurfaced in his life after twenty-five years, but strangely enough, her reemergence serves a purpose. Though he is clearly not himself, they talk frequently, and I soon confirm that their suggestive storytelling is leading to phone sex. The lady in question seems to need this as much as Nicky.

My initial reaction is, *What is she doing? Doesn't she realize that he is ill?* Then I take a deep breath and accept that there is no real harm in this fantasy life that is playing out on the telephone. I go back to *there is no blame / there is no shame.* I know, in the overall scheme of things, this is doing more good than harm, and I can live with it. What is so extraordinary about this bizarre turn of events is that Nicky trusts me and tells me everything, and for this I remain grateful. Mercifully, neither of us feels guilt about what is needed . . . that's just life. Absurdly, we all win.

SEPTEMBER 2019

- September 11: More confusion and obsessive behavior are setting in. Nicky starts talking in the middle of his thought, and it's hard to follow. He gets an idée fixe and won't leave it alone.

- September 12: His weight in September is fluctuating between 102 and 106.

- September 13: Nicky falls on the street walking alone on his return from the post office one-and-a-half blocks from our home. He comes in confused with a bruised face and a black eye; he can't tell me if anyone helped him or exactly where he fell. Even though the birthday card he purchased at the post office is in his hand, he cannot remember where he has been or what he bought or for whom he bought it. He is visibly shaken, and we resolve together that I will accompany him on any future excursions outside the apartment building. No more trips outside alone.

- September 14: Still shaken and tired, with a full-blown black eye, he remains a bit foggy. He has a family visit with children, which is always a great tonic, but cuts out in the early afternoon for a two-hour nap.

- September 15: He is very tired and rests all day.

- September 16: Nicky is still a bit foggy and having trouble remembering his schedule.

- September 17: Today is a bit better; he is brighter and not as tired or foggy.

- September 19: We visit our primary care physician, Dr. John Cahill, whom we both love and trust. He is very pleased with Nicky's walking and progress with physical therapy and also happy with the speech therapy results. It is music to my hears when Cahill instructs no more unaccompanied stair climbing for exercise.

- September 30: Nicky has lunch with a friend and falls on the way home. Our friend tells me Nicky does not want me to know. Later Nicky tells me that people are tripping on the street. When I ask, "Did you trip?" he says, "No." I just let it go.

This is a moment I have dreaded, the moment when I have to say that it is no longer possible for Nicky to leave the apartment unaccompanied. His independence is his trademark, and now I have to curb that too. Instead of saying "you can't," which is always a red flag, I turn it into something delightful, saying, "From now on, let's plan on doing everything together. You just let me know when you want to go somewhere, and I will rearrange my schedule to do it. It's going to be fun to do more together, after all, we are always wanting to, so let's just do it." Nicky's initial reaction is one of relief, but I know it will not stay that way. Independence is too much a part of his DNA.

OCTOBER 2019

- October 1–2: Nicky shows lots of anger at me and at the speech therapist. Confusion is high and he is very foggy. Late at night on October 2, his legs are bothering him—hurting and itchy; he knocks over a whole tumbler of water at 2:00 a.m., not the most conducive hour for cleanup; it's getting harder for me to keep calm and keep balanced and upbeat; Nicky did not have a nap during the day, and that also creates anxiety.
- October 15–17: I am in London for business, and my brother, Louis, comes to stay with Nicky, but Louis gets a severe virus (mercifully Nicky did not get it); Nicky complains that while I am away, people are taking charge, and he is also angry that I left all the vital information (travel

itinerary, emergency numbers, etc.) with my brother and not with him. He begins misinterpreting things that are said (either mishearing or hallucinating); however, he does very well with the pill chart I leave for him, successfully checking off each box.

- October 19–20: I am now back home, and Nicky is very tired, angry, and still mishearing what's being said. He is sleeping a great deal—throughout the night until 9:00 a.m. and also napping during the day.
- During October, he is having very active dream activity and needs constant assurances that they are not real, finding it hard to differentiate between dream and reality.
- His hands are shaking more than usual, especially as he sleeps.
- During waking hours, his right foot is dragging more.

It is now clear to me that I will not be taking any more business trips. It's too upsetting for Nicky, and it's not fair to place that responsibility on someone else.

NOVEMBER 2019

- November 18: Now there is anger at not being able to go out alone. Nicky announces that he is going by himself to the new Upper West Side Copy Center location on Seventy-Second Street, five blocks away from our home; I ask if he could wait until the following day for me to accompany him, and he does.
- November 20: Nicky tells the physical therapist about wanting to go out alone; unsolicited, she says, "No, listen to Mary Lou."
- November 21: Nicky calls me in the middle of a business meeting I am attending at Lincoln Center: Without

warning me in advance and fully aware of our agreement, he has gone out alone to walk around the block, but on his return, he can't get his key to work in the door of our main apartment. He could, however, get into my office, which is across the hall from the apartment, and is calling my cell phone from my landline; I tell him to go to the lobby and ask the doorman to help him. He does, the doorman is wonderful, and all is fine. When I come home, I am angry inside, fighting to keep my outside cool. I calmly say we will discuss this with Dr. Cahill as I am not going to fight; but I will never compromise on his safety—that is nonnegotiable.

- November 23: Nicky awakes with hallucinations and bad dreams; it's hard for him to tell dreams from reality, and my job is to calm him and bring back a sense of reality. He keeps misplacing his glasses and diary. There is a lot of anger coming from him.

- November 24: At a dinner with friends, Nicky is really out of it, making very little sense and speaking in sentence fragments, not able to finish a sentence. He is actually falling asleep at the table. There's a look of blankness that accompanies this. This is the worst he's been in public.

- We drive to Ogunquit, Maine, to our favorite resort, The Cliff House, for a three-day Thanksgiving excursion with my sister, Angel. Nicky is tired but fine and receives lots of positive reinforcement. Familiar places seem to work; new places don't.

That dinner with friends was a turning point, a real preview of coming attractions, and it is upsetting to witness. It is becoming clear that this roller-coaster behavior is going to become part of the LBD cycle as life progresses. The major challenge is the unpredictability . . . you never see it coming, there is no warning, it is just there.

DECEMBER 2019

- December 4: Following a delightful lunch with a chef friend and after we return home, Nicky comes into my office to ask how to put his jacket on the hanger, he can't figure it out.

- There is general confusion, not completing thoughts, searching for words, and being very tired.

- Week of December 8: Nicky is needing more support to stand from a seated position; more confusion is creeping in. He is not hearing clearly even with his hearing aid in. He still maintains a good walking momentum; he takes almost two hours to shower and dress, which I let him do as it's a sense of accomplishment for him; buttoning his shirt is very slow; he has trouble putting on a jacket without help; using the zipper of his jacket is challenging (I do it most of the time); his right foot is beginning to drag even more and extend slightly to the side.

- December 14: Nicky weighs in at an alarming 98.6 pounds, and he is disturbed by this, as am I; he's been averaging about 102 to 103.

- He is saying that I am not doing enough for him, that I am always occupied with other things. While I am sure this is exactly what he is feeling, he is also absolutely correct that I am continuing to work while taking care of him, and it's two full-time jobs. It is also true that my work helps me to keep my sanity and my positive focus.

- I speak with Nicky's sister Lucy and tell her that reaching out to him once a month is not enough; I need her more involved for him, and he needs to see his family, not just mine.

- December 16: Nicky is back to 100 pounds, he is very tired and weak and sleeping a lot.

- Christmas: What a wonderful and positive time as we stay for two nights at the home of my sister, Angel, in Morristown, New Jersey. (God bless Uber for providing an easy trip.) My brother, Louis, arrives from Florida to join us. It's wonderful that my brother and sister are so supportive of Nicky and me. We have a glorious family Christmas with lots of laughter and love.

- December 28: Nicky falls on the street while I am holding him. He is making noises again about going out alone and having his independence taken away. He speaks regularly now with his lady friend, but mercifully he never actually sees her as she lives too far away and Zoom videoconferencing confuses him. She continues to feed him with sexual fantasies by phone; he says he needs sex or this tantalizing substitute. It comforts him and, while it's annoying to me, I figure it's harmless and a small price to pay for his contentment. I also think it empowers him to be his own person with someone who has nothing to do with me and doesn't even know me.

- December 30: Today I gave Nicky a two-hour window to shower and dress before meeting friends for lunch. When I came across the hall from my office to get him, he has showered but is not dressed. I lose my cool and agitatedly hurry him along by dressing him so that we can be on time for our lunch date. After my frenzy of getting him ready, I am so sorry that I made him feel bad. I need to work harder to keep calm in these situations. He already feels bad enough, he doesn't need me to compound the situation. He looked at me with tears in his eyes and for the first time said, "*I am sick.*" It broke my heart.

- There has been lots of diarrhea, and he fears it; I have succeeded in getting him to wear Depends (disposable underpants for incontinence), which he seems to like now, and it makes him feel more confident; he had resisted using them for six months, but now the timing is right.
- Physical therapy continues to be very helpful, and speech therapy is moderately helpful; both are concluding.

I am facing a major dilemma. While I have talked several times in this narrative about sexual needs as generally regards LBD and specifically regards Nicky, I also made a solemn pledge to Nicky to help him keep his dignity, as he asked me to do when he was diagnosed back in March 2019. This is something I take very seriously. As I said earlier, my energy has limits, but for Nicky I know sex is still a very real part of the very little that he can control. I will myself to detach from the situation, sometimes pretending not to notice what is going on, other times deliberately helping to dial the lady friend's phone number when Nicky is not able. Why? Because it helps him, and it helps me to see the relief on his face. I tell myself that it means nothing but physical release, and it's true because Nicky always tells me about the encounters. He even tells me that she lately has been insisting that she is better for him, could take better care of him than I can, and that someday they will be together. These comments inwardly make me see red, but it's a relief to know that Nicky realizes this is a bunch of bunk and tells me so. What is important is that he is content and still in charge of this area of his life.

JANUARY 2020

- A positive influence and source of great happiness to start the new year is our beautiful godson who lights up a room and adores Nicky. Needless to say, Nicky adores him right back. On January 2, we arrange an outing with godson Andrew and his mom/our niece Amanda to the Rockefeller Center Christmas tree and have a joyful dinner together. Nicky is happy but exhausted and sleeps the entire next day. My feeling is that giving Nicky happy times is important, and if the price is sleeping for a day, why not?

- Nicky is a showman, the rock 'n' roller has never left the room. When we have a lunch or dinner with friends, he makes a real effort to marshal all his energy to be the old Nicky. He then pays the price by sleeping a great deal, sometimes even all of the following day, which I do not discourage. This is happening more and more.

- January 18: Nicky says, "I don't trust you." This is hurtful to me; I begin to realize when "Lewy" is talking. The mistrust subsides after a few hours.

- January 19: Miraculously we have a five-hour lunch at home with wonderful and stimulating friends. The old Nicky is present and loves the interaction.

- January 20: The Metropolitan Museum of Art has a Félix Vallotton exhibit that Nicky wants to see. It's a small exhibit, and during the hour we are there, we view it twice and then go to The Met dining room for lunch. It's like the old days. He also loved going to MoMA on January 14 for a members' evening to see the newly renovated museum space. Right now, art in small doses with special exhibits is positive and stimulating, especially followed by a meal to discuss what we have seen.

- January 26: This is a rough patch—Nicky is angry and suspicious. I have triggered trust issues by replacing an old, dirty, throw rug in Nicky's art studio space without asking permission, a total mistake on my part. He admitted it was right to get rid of it, but said I should have asked him first, and he is 100 percent correct (lesson learned).

So many things during January seemed hopeful and positive. The socializing was wonderful, and the museum trips brought back old, joyful times. Throughout our life together, we would frequently spend time in museums all over the world, following these excursions with a lunch or dinner or cocktails. One of our favorite late Saturday afternoon activities, following long walks and gallery exploring, was going to an elegant New York hotel bar for drinks and conversation, just the two of us.

FEBRUARY 2020

- Week of February 9: Nicky works on another portrait of our godson, Andrew. It takes everything out of him, but the result is vintage Nicky.
- February 15: We attend godson Andrew's third birthday party at a kids' center in Westchester for twenty children; this is followed by a family dinner at Nicky's sister Lucy's home. I should have guessed that it would be too much for Nicky as he fell fast asleep at the dinner table. Afterward Nicky said, "This is probably the last time for this type of activity." Even though we Ubered out and back, it's now just too much. I am glad he is realizing this.
- February 16: We attend a birthday party for a close friend with twelve guests at a lovely Midtown restaurant, and Nicky does really well.

- February 17: Even though it's two consecutive evenings, generally not a good idea, we have dinner in our neighborhood with very understanding friends whose calm works like a charm, and Nicky loves this evening.
- Week of February 18: It is no surprise that total exhaustion sets in with minor hallucinating.
- Nicky loves to exercise, he always has, and feels much better after, albeit very tired. I try to get him out once a day for a short walk, sometimes stopping for lunch.
- Movies and concerts no longer work: Nicky gets into a theater, falls asleep, and then wakes up disoriented; this is not a good combo.

GENERAL OBSERVATIONS MARKING ONE YEAR SINCE THE OFFICIAL LBD DIAGNOSIS:

- Nicky's weight is up and averaging 104–106; he's eating well.
- His fatigue is increasing, and he sleeps a great deal during the day and through the night.
- He is sad that he has no autonomy regarding leaving the house unaccompanied.
- There is sadness creeping in about his condition in general, and I hate seeing my upbeat Nicky so unhappy.
- His right foot is noticeably dragging.
- His speech is much slower, and he takes more time to develop a thought and articulate it. This from the man whose quick wit and intricate storytelling were his signature.
- All activity is slower—walking, dressing, talking, thinking, reacting.
- Dressing is a challenge, and he often needs help to figure out what to wear and how to put it on; zippers are especially challenging.

The limitations are beginning to clearly define themselves, and while I see them, I wait for Nicky to make his own observations. I then agree with him and change the pattern to accommodate his energy levels. I will keep everything moving for as long as Nicky is comfortable, never pushing beyond his capability. He is the driver, and I hold the road map and can change the route for him at any time.

MARCH 2020

- March 16: This date marks the beginning of a new way of living. COVID-19 has struck, and Nicky is periodically confused by it. He really doesn't understand why I am so insistent on hand washing and being extra vigilant. It's an ongoing challenge and causes arguments. If his safety is not being compromised, I can relax about anything. The minute his safety is in question, I become a pit bull.
- Week of March 22: Nicky experiences two bouts of massive diarrhea. The first time, I wake to a running shower at 5:00 a.m.; Nicky had soiled himself and has meticulously cleaned up both the site of the accident as best he can and himself. Even though he wears Depends day and night, the bed is soiled, and I am commandeering our laundry room at 6:00 a.m. (thank goodness there is a laundry room on every floor). On the second occasion, I am prepared with pads for the bed (like they use in hospitals, placed on top of the sheet), and it saves the day.
- March 27: Following a strong argument about his safety, Nicky draws a picture of the two of us hugging in the sunlight with masks on, with the cartoon bubble reading: "You're only trying to help me! I'm so sorry!" This was the very last picture he ever drew, and he even signed it with his signature Z.

- During the March and April lockdown, so much has changed because of COVID. I find the following happening with Nicky:

  ► Lots of mood swings and finding a lot of fault with me.

  ► He's increasingly finicky about food, because he is afraid of diarrhea. I keep trying to assure him it is the disease and not the food. I try to make the parallel that, just as his nose constantly runs because of the LBD, the same is true for diarrhea as an LBD symptom.

  ► Walks and sunlight and fresh air are helpful, and we are very careful not to overdo it.

  ► Still being negatively influenced by his long-distance phone friend, I can tell when he has had a conversation with her, as he gets a bit mean-spirited with me and frequently says that I make her uncomfortable because I am abrupt with her. She is clearly feeding him negative thoughts. This begins to come to a natural end when, in April, Nicky is not able to make much sense and is difficult to follow, and the phone lady just stops talking to him. So much for her compassion. When there is clearly nothing in it any longer for her, she is finished, and her cruelty toward him is unconscionable. Mercifully, he doesn't seem to miss her calls.

  ► He sleeps a lot more during daytime, and also sleeps all night through.

  ► His weight is between 99 and 103 pounds.

  ► He is eating well.

  ► He is very clean and fastidious.

  ► Most of the time, he is sweet and caring.

> ▸ He knows he is having more cognitive problems and often asks the person with whom he is speaking if he is making sense.
> ▸ Sometimes he makes sense and is brilliant.
> ▸ Other times, I cannot follow what he is saying.

I guess if you are patient, the right solutions will appear. While I did nothing to end Nicky's joy in telephoning with his lady friend, when the sledding got rough and she realized she couldn't control him even in his fragile state, she just abruptly cut out. What I noticed was that what might have begun months earlier as a release of sorts was becoming a source of great agitation for Nicky as she began to admonish him when something wasn't to her liking. As Nicky's protector and spouse, I walk a fine line and only want him to be safe and comfortable. It was such a blessing when it resolved itself and she was out of the picture for good.

APRIL 2020

- Hallucinations are now prevalent: bugs crawling on the bathroom wall, bunny in the bedroom, person standing behind me.
- His voice is hoarse, very soft with no volume.
- Nicky finds it increasingly difficult to express thoughts; he knows what he wants to convey but cannot get the words out.
- He gets angry when I don't understand and ask for more information.
- He sleeps a great deal, both day and night.
- There are a few days of evening incontinence with loose bowels and two accidents.
- He has difficulty following a conversation and comes into the discussion with non sequiturs.

- He doesn't always understand what is happening with the COVID virus.
- He bristles at my directions to keep him safe, especially the hand washing after walks.
- He has very limited ability with Zoom videoconferencing; he thinks the people on the screen are in the next room; he cannot be heard as his voice is too weak.
- It is interesting that he is better at WhatsApp video with one person, especially our three-year-old godson, Andrew, and our friends of more than fifty years who call regularly from Lucca, Italy.

I am seeing a marked decline during April. Everything is beginning to slowly break down, and the isolation due to COVID is making us cocoon more and more. Now is when I probably would have brought in some caregiving help, but with COVID it's not possible. Thank goodness I am blessed with a great deal of energy and seem to be able to handle what is and hopefully what is coming. Nicky is just delighted that it's the two of us 24/7 and is content to be with just me. Our trusted and beautiful neighbor friends come in to share a meal every now and then, and while Nicky loves the wife, he seems to get easily annoyed with her husband. Nicky takes exception when what he is enduring is dismissed or ignored as if everything is fine. He is extremely sensitive. I become very careful about what energy I allow to be around him. He is sensitive to energy, and I want as toxic-free an environment as I can create for him.

MAY 2020
- Early May, his weight is hovering between 97 and 101 pounds.
- Every morning, Nicky is now weighing under 100, and it's alarming to us both.

- He is confused most of the time.
- He continues to bristle at my insistence on hand washing and on not touching others.
- Being affable and tactile, he always wants to hug someone or wants to shake hands and still cannot understand why he can't.
- Hallucinations and bad dreams are frequent, and it's important to reassure him that he is safe, protected, and above all loved.
- It's the first Saturday in May, and Nicky gets out of the shower crying and saying, "I am dying and I know it." This is a huge admission for Nicky who has consistently said, "I am going to beat this." My response while crying with him is, "Yes, we are all going to die, just not today."
- He asks, "Can I trust you?" and I ask back, "Do you think you can?" His answer is, "Yes," and I respond, "And you can."
- Conversations are difficult as he makes little sense.
- Week of May 20: Rough week, bad dreams and hallucinations, everything more negative than positive, he fatigues easily.
- Nicky awoke one morning this week at 5:00 a.m. agitated about something I couldn't understand.
- He had a few days of nausea and dizziness and was afraid to eat too much.
- He was a frightening 95.8 pounds.
- I have to be with him more.
- He can still walk, but more than forty-five minutes does not work; one day we walked for more than an hour, and it was clearly too much.
- I have to work at keeping an even tone of love and support, even when I am told by Nicky that *I am the crazy one.*

- May 23: He weighs 94.3 pounds, has no appetite, is slightly dizzy, and there is still a bit of nausea but without vomiting this time.
- Nicky is becoming negative and snappish.
- May 25: He weighs 93 pounds . . . ugh, I don't know what to do. He experiences great fatigue, asks for pasta for lunch, and then goes right to sleep.
- Nicky rises in the morning about 10:00 a.m. It takes one or two hours to get ready. He eats his first meal of the day around 11:30; he grazes in the afternoon on crackers and cottage cheese and yogurt; he sleeps more; he rises for dinner around 7:00 p.m.; he falls asleep right after dinner.
- He is sleeping fifteen to twenty hours per day.
- May 24: He has no voice, no sound, cannot talk.
- Privately, I am concerned that it's nearing the end, and Nicky has been referencing this feeling independent of me.
- May 27: A good, positive day, and we are looking forward to going to our apartment building roof deck and seeing a few neighbor friends at a safe distance. Nicky is eating well today.

Such a set of mixed emotions. My beautiful Nicky is now entering the realm of existing from day to day, rather than living as he always did. There is so little for him to enjoy. Our ritual of holding each other is still in play, and we often go to sleep holding hands. I watch him sleep, wondering where he is and what he is experiencing. I know that in his lucid moments he is aware of everything that is happening to him. (After Nicky died, I had this confirmed when I found a poem that Nicky wrote around this time. In chapter 48, Nicky describes through this poem that the invasive stranger entered our home, wouldn't leave, and was periodically taking over.) It must be frightening for him. For me, it is heartbreaking to see my extraordinary life partner leaving me a little bit more every day. Nicky is both absent and present at the same time . . . a strange dichotomy.

JUNE 2020

- We had an incident: Nicky was in his studio, which is down the hall from our apartment, obsessing about finding something, I can't even remember what it was. We looked in every closet and drawer and nook and cranny. When we couldn't find what he was looking for, he wanted to repeat the whole process, at which point I firmly said *please, no, we have done that.* He got very upset with me, and we went back to our apartment where I made him a cup of tea and left him sitting in the living room to calm down. When I returned in about one hour, he was sound asleep in a chair. I gently woke him and asked if he wanted to rest in the bedroom. He couldn't stand up, so I lifted him to his feet. Then he couldn't figure out how to walk, so I gently instructed him to put one foot forward, then the next, all the while holding his hands and walking backward with him coming toward me. We made it to the bedroom, and he slept soundly.

- Sleeping continues to be excessive. Nicky now rises around 11:30 a.m. to eat, then showers, and is often so tired after showering that he sleeps again.

- We try to walk every day and average between four to five times a week, varying from twenty to forty minutes each time. We walk very slowly, him holding on to me, and he seems to like doing this.

- June 7: Nicky's seventy-seventh birthday. He enjoys all the good wishes coming his way via cards, telephone calls, Skype sessions, WhatsApp videos.

- June 9: Nicky has trouble getting on his jeans. He gets stuck halfway between falling off the bed where his arms are supporting him and sitting on the floor where his feet are. What he is unable to figure out is how to get back to sitting on the edge of the bed or lowering himself to sit on the floor. When I come in, he is thoroughly confused, hanging onto the bed for dear life and not knowing how to either get back to sitting or safely lower himself to the floor. He is so rigid that I have to lift him up and place him on the bed so that we can put his jeans on.

- June 15: Today is a day that I have been dreading. I purchase the "chair with wheels" and tell Nicky that it is a gift from our doctor, John Cahill. What I know is that no matter how much he needs the help of a wheelchair, he will reject it if he knows I purchased it. And so, I choose a little white lie instead to accomplish what I know has to happen.

- A few days later when Dr. John Cahill makes a house call, I tell him about the wheelchair and how I got Nicky to accept it. I didn't want him to be surprised when Nicky thanks him, which Nicky of course does.

- John was surprised at how quickly the LBD had progressed. Thanks to COVID, he had not actually seen Nicky for five months.

What a beautiful day Nicky's birthday was. Love poured in from all over the world. It was as if the universe knew that this would be his last birthday. Since Nicky so loved being outdoors in the beautiful weather we were having, and since we had several times barely made it home from our walks, I knew it was time for a wheelchair and had to find a way to get Nicky to accept it. I remembered how adamant he had been last year about not wanting to use a wheelchair at the airport. Thus I felt just fine about telling him that the "chair with wheels," always mindful not to use the word *wheelchair* in his presence, was a gift from Dr. Cahill.

On our first outing with the chair, Nicky and I both pushed it out of the building. I waited until we were a few blocks away from our building in a small park with a few benches around and said that I was a bit tired and wanted to rest for a minute. I sat on a bench and suggested that Nicky might like to just take a seat in the comfortable new chair, which he did. When it was time to go, I asked if he would like to push it again or might he like to stay seated and give it a spin to try it out. He agreed to stay seated and off we went down to the Hudson River.

It was a glorious day, and Nicky was enjoying the scenery and the air without a care in the world. I couldn't have been happier watching the delight it brought him. On our way back, we stopped in another small park a block from our home. I asked if, when we got closer to our building, might he like to get out of the chair and walk into the building. His answer was "maybe." As we got close to home, Nicky made no effort to signal that he wanted out of the chair, and I didn't ask again. Into the building we rolled, and Nicky was just fine, head held high and dignity intact.

This was a rough month. There were days when I was the two Mary Lous, meaning he was seeing me in duplicate. And there were days when Nicky didn't know who I was. I would ask, "Nicky, do you know who I am," and he would very calmly say, "No, but that's all right." He clearly knows the sound of my voice, and it must be calming; and he knows my touch, so he isn't frightened. He also has no fear of death because he believes in God and in an afterlife. He believes in Heaven.

JULY 2020

- Very early July brings on Nicky's aggressive behavior and anxiousness. I am advised to make sure that all the visible knives in the kitchen are stored safely out of sight. This is a precaution that all LBD caregivers are given in case anything gets violent, which it can. Mercifully, this doesn't happen to us. Dr. Cahill puts Nicky on a low dose of Seroquel, which makes him very agitated almost immediately. With Nicky, it has just the opposite effect of the calming it is supposed to induce. This sometimes happens with people with LBD. We have to wean Nicky off, but the aggression remains.

- July 7: Niece Amanda and godson Andrew come for lunch, but Nicky is able to stay with them only for an hour. He stops eating that day, and I know it's time to arrange for hospice help. I check on Nicky who is peacefully sleeping, before going back across the hall to my office to call Dr. Cahill, who helps me make hospice arrangements. While I am busy processing these arrangements, Nicky has awakened and unbeknownst to me has had a major, unusual bowel accident, trailing sticky, clay-like feces from the bedroom to the bathroom, through the hallway into the living room, and straight into the kitchen, not to mention sticking to him like glue. Strength kicks in when you need it, and very calmly I first get Nicky into the shower to clean him up. That accomplished, I leave him sitting quietly in the bathroom bundled in a fluffy towel as I strip and remake the bed so that he can comfortably rest while I spend the next four hours cleaning everything else. All the while, it is important to keep Nicky calm, repeating the mantra "you are safe, you are protected, you are loved." I let him know that these things happen, there's nothing to worry about, everything is fine, it's no problem. What I recognize is that this is the beginning of the end. The body is having one last massive expulsion of feces that resembles meconium (a baby's first poop) before beginning to shut down for good.

- July 9: Nicky has not been eating for two days, and now he stops drinking anything. Hospice comes to evaluate, and we are accepted immediately. They know Nicky does not have long to live. They deliver their standard "end of life" kit, which, in addition to morphine, contains Haldol, a drug that should *never* be used by anyone with LBD. They also offer oxygen, which I decline. Nicky's breathing is not labored, and I am afraid that introducing oxygen, especially as it will need to be attached to his face, will just confuse and frighten him. When I check with Dr. Cahill, I am happy to hear him confirm I did the right thing.

  Now is the time to rally the family and close friends for one last goodbye, COVID be damned! Late afternoon, with everyone gathered, they go to the bedroom one at a time. With everyone now reconvened in the living room, I hear my name being called. When I go to see Nicky, he actually asks to be wheeled into the living room to see everyone together and miraculously makes one last appearance. Not only does he see everyone, but with his signature smile, he says a last goodbye to each and every one by name. He then tells me he is tired and wants to go back to bed.

- July 10: A few more visitors.
- July 11: It is 5:00 a.m., and knowing how Nicky loves to be clean, I ask if he would like me to shave and shower him. The shaving is easy, but where I get the strength to get him into the shower without dropping him, and

then succeed in getting him out of the shower (it's an old-fashioned tub where you have to step up and over), I will never know, although I am helped by the fact that he weighs only eighty-nine pounds. A few final visitors, including my dear friend Mary Beth Peil, who stays for the duration. She doesn't want me to face the end alone and knows me so well after fifty years that she is right there if I need, and in the wings when I don't. A priest does last rights at 1:30 p.m. via speakerphone.

- July 12–13: No more visitors. What I realized yesterday was that as long as anyone but me was in the room, Nicky, the consummate entertainer, felt obliged to be the host. All goodbyes have been said, and quiet and calm are now needed to allow Nicky the freedom to process peacefully to the other side. He is still trying to get up to use the bathroom, but his legs won't support him. Keeping him calm and clean and comfortable with morphine, I sleep by his side—as I have for thirty-seven years—watching and waiting . . .

CHAPTER 50

Last Goodbye

If the heart has devoted itself to love, there is not a single inch of emptiness.

—*Mary Oliver*

Our hearts are breaking as together we accept the truth: In this lifetime, we are losing each other . . .

Your body is shutting down. Even though we are still in deep COVID lockdown, family and close friends come to say their last goodbyes. I call a priest and manage to arrange last rites for you over the phone. I'm thankful my best friend, Mary Beth Peil, has come to stay and help us. A few days later, on Bastille Day, July 14, 2020, at 10:20 a.m., you quietly let go of this world, your dignity intact.

With a heavy heart and with Mary Beth's help, I prepare you for the next life, dressing you in the stylish clothes you loved. Then, in a last private hour together, I thank you for our wonderful life together, repeating aloud your wise words: "We have had a great run, we cannot be sad." With a final kiss at the front door, I whisper, "I love you, safe journey . . ."

I miss you so much every day, my beloved Nicky, but am comforted knowing that you are *home* now, and at peace.

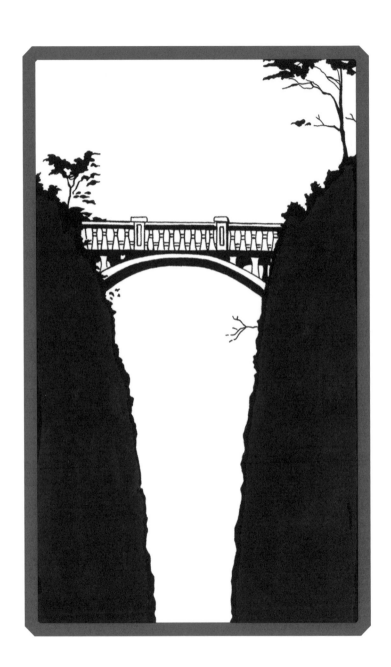

The Ending

2020

Death
You surround us
You circle us
And then, expected or not,
You take
And we have no recourse
But to surrender.

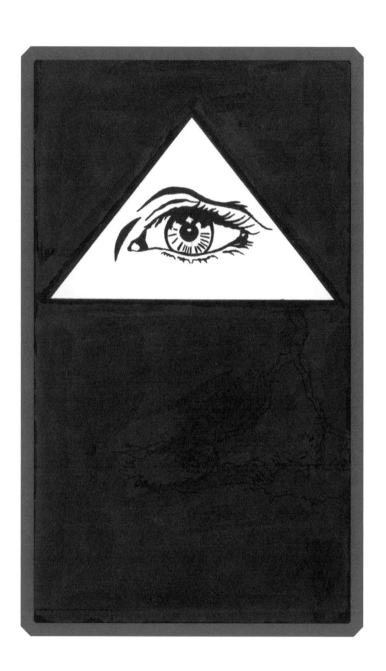

Waves

2021

A wave washes over me
Like a blanket of sadness,
And, for a moment,
Takes my breath away.
Then I remember his words,
"We have had a great run,
we cannot be sad,"
And peace returns.
Alone again
Now in sunlight,
Until the next wave . . .

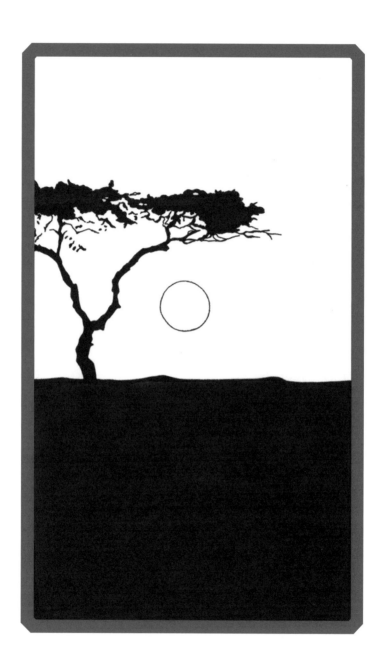

The Prayer

Love never disappears, for death is a nonevent.
I have merely retired to the room next door.
You and I are the same; what we were for each other, we still are.
Speak to me as you always have, do not use a different tone,
    do not be sad.
Continue to laugh at what made us laugh.
Smile and think of me.
Life means what it has always meant.
The link is not severed.
Why should I be out of your soul if I am out of your sight?
I will wait for you, I am not here, but just on the other side
    of this path.
You see, all is well.

—Saint Augustine

Help and Resources for Lewy Body and Related Dementia

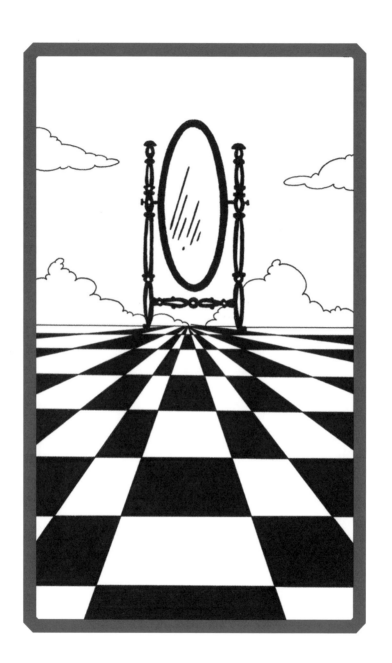

Meet "Lewy":
An Accessible Introduction to
Lewy Body Dementia

Welcome to the elusive world of Lewy body dementia (sometimes called Lewy body disease), where the saying goes, "If you've met one person with LBD, you've met *one* person with LBD."

Dementia in general is a scary word, and it's a big umbrella for many types of brain declines especially as people get older. Early onset dementia can happen to people in their forties. We all know someone with some type of dementia, and it's heartbreaking. Simply put, dementia is the brain misfiring in ways that interfere with daily function, that is, thinking and acting.

In this general overview, my goal is to get the reader specifically acquainted with LBD. What exactly is it? My simple answer: LBD is a nasty and cruel disease, a complex and challenging brain disorder that takes you on a merciless roller-coaster ride, with the only off switch currently being death. First it takes away your executive function and cognitive ability but, just to confuse the issue, gives both functions back from time to time so that you can periodically be 100 percent yourself. And people suffering with LBD are very much aware of what's happening, especially on their good days. It's difficult to diagnose, there is no slowing it down, and no medication that can stop it. LBD is a neurodegenerative disease, which in simple terms means it's incurable and debilitating and results in progressive degeneration and death of nerve cells. LBD comes with a host of physical, cognitive, and behavioral symptoms. Movement becomes a problem along with mental functioning, and a person's abilities to walk, speak, swallow, and accomplish even simple tasks are ultimately affected.

Lewy body dementia is an umbrella term that refers to two diagnoses: dementia with Lewy bodies (DLB) and Parkinson's disease dementia (PDD). Though the diagnostic criteria for DLB and PDD differ, the associated symptoms are largely the same. I wish I could give you a definitive checklist, preferably in order of appearance. But, alas, LBD doesn't behave in an orderly or predictable way; one size does not fit all. Here are some of the signs that you might see:

- Cognitive issues: A person with LBD will generally show a continued decline in cognition (for example, slowness in retrieving thoughts or losing train of thought), judgment, problem-solving, multitasking, planning, thinking, and fluctuations in alertness. As executive function decreases, memory itself starts to fade—short-term memory first, and long-term memory toward the end (the shorthand is "first in, last out").
- Movement issues (Parkinsonism): Signs may include a shuffling gait, tremors, balance problems, difficulty walking, stooped posture, loss of coordination, impaired depth perception, slowness in walking and moving in general, and stiffness or rigidity in the legs and arms. The hands may also become weak and stiff.
- Some people will show symptoms of both cognitive and movement problems within the first year. Others may have difficulty with movement first and dementia later on, indicating Parkinson's disease dementia.

- Hallucinations: Common images are of children and small animals. Sometimes there are auditory hallucinations; and misidentification of people and objects can be typical in LBD.
- REM sleep behavior disorder (acting out your dreams physically while asleep) or restless leg syndrome can be early signs of LBD.
- People with LBD tend to be sensitive to medications, often having harmful and/or paradoxical reactions; be especially cautious with "first generation" antipsychotic drugs.
- Fluctuations are a key element. At times people tend to be more alert and awake, while other times they are more confused, sedate, or irritable.
- Depression, delusions, anger, anxiety, apathy, paranoia, agitation, and daytime sleepiness are LBD symptoms.
- Other symptoms can include fainting due to low blood pressure, frequent falls, sensitivity to heat and cold, incontinence, constipation.
- Lesser-known LBD symptoms may include a constantly dripping nose, loss of smell, and handwriting that gets smaller and smaller.
- Some experience Capgras syndrome, a delusional belief that a person has been replaced by an imposter.
- The general thinking is that LBD has a lifespan from diagnosis to death of five to eight years, but occasionally it is less than two and often considerably more than ten.
- According to the Mayo Clinic, a diagnosis of LBD requires a progressive decline in the ability to think, as well as at least two of the following: fluctuating alertness and thinking function; repeated visual hallucinations; Parkinsonian symptoms; REM sleep behavior disorder.

- The main differences between Alzheimer's disease and LBD are that people with Alzheimer's disease are much more likely to have memory impairment and face a less severe loss of executive function in the disease's early stages.
- While there is currently no definitive test to confirm Lewy body dementia, the following can be helpful tools to support an LBD diagnosis:
  - ▶ REM sleep test
  - ▶ DaTscan
  - ▶ PET scan
  - ▶ MRI
  - ▶ Skin biopsy that is highly sensitive and specific for LBD (CND Life Sciences)
  - ▶ Amprion SYNTAP Biomarker Test (spinal fluid test)
- Note: *Always consult with a neurologist.* A movement disorder neurologist can be particularly helpful regarding LBD.

What is actually happening in the brain when one has LBD? In lay terms, abnormal protein deposits known as Lewy bodies (unhealthy alpha-synuclein is the main component in Lewy bodies, which are named after their discoverer, Dr. Friedrich Lewy, a German neurologist) manifest inside the brain cells, clog the cells, and the cells die. These chemical changes in the brain can lead to problems with thinking, movement, behavior, and mood. LBD seems to occur randomly, and no one knows the cause. More men than women seem to be affected. LBD progresses more rapidly than Alzheimer's disease and typically begins in one's sixties or seventies. And it is possible to have mixed dementia; for example, Alzheimer's disease can coexist with Lewy body dementia.

Early on in my acquaintanceship with LBD, very few people knew what I was referencing when I mentioned that my beloved husband, Nicky Zann, had been diagnosed with the disease. Anecdotally, when I told people about it, nine out of ten had never heard of it, and among the people who had, an even smaller number knew anything about it, including how to spell "Lewy." One prominent CEO of a major arts institution in New York City told me that she spent more than an hour online trying to research the disease but couldn't figure out how to spell it.

When Nicky died in 2020, I knew my mission was to eradicate two phrases: "Lewy what?" and "How do you spell that?" Nicky's struggle—along with that of so many others—had to count, and something meaningful had to be done to advance the cause.

Facts that bear repeating:

- Lewy body dementia is the second most common form of progressive dementia after Alzheimer's disease and affects more than 1.4 million Americans. It is widely misdiagnosed, as it can mimic Alzheimer's disease, Parkinson's disease, or a psychiatric disorder.
- LBD is a neurodegenerative brain disease in which one size does not fit all, making it very hard to diagnose and, once diagnosed, difficult to treat and currently impossible to cure.
- More people have LBD than amyotrophic lateral sclerosis (ALS), muscular dystrophy, and cerebral palsy *combined*.
- More people have LBD than are HIV positive.
- Among those who have suffered from and lost the battle with LBD, in addition to my husband, Nicky Zann, are Tom Seaver, Dina Merrill, Estelle Getty, Casey Kasem, and Frank Corsaro. Through autopsy, it was discovered that Robin Williams also had LBD. And who knows how many others have been misdiagnosed?

These facts need to be more widely known. Key to opening the door to LBD is awareness—for health care professionals and the general public alike. As I have mentioned before, my lifeline during Nicky's illness was the Lewy Body Dementia Resource Center. After Nicky passed, Founder and Executive Director Norma Loeb invited me to join the board of directors of LBDRC, knowing that its mission of "bringing awareness, supporting with love" is totally aligned with my own.

When you hear the words *Lewy body dementia*, most people become immobilized and don't know where to turn. I regret to say that many doctors, while brilliant at diagnosis, are not particularly helpful beyond that. Resources and assistance for people with LBD and their families still remain extremely limited. The Lewy Body Dementia Resource Center was founded in 2016 to provide needed resources and support for people with LBD and their loved ones who are their main caregivers. This support includes the only *live* helpline in the United States (833-LBD-LINE), available 365 days a year, along with regular support groups for both caregivers and those with LBD. The LBDRC website (www.lewybodyresourcecenter.org) offers valuable information about neurologists, physical and occupational therapists with knowledge of LBD, adult day care programs, house call programs, hospice agencies, meal deliveries, transportation, music, art and movement therapies, as well as all aspects of caregiving specifically for New York, Florida, and California. Information about neurologists and other knowledgeable physicians is now listed on the LBDRC website for every state in the United States as well as twenty-five additional countries.

You are not alone! The daily struggles and sometimes horrors of living with LBD are real for you and your loved one. I want to emphasize the importance of love, dignity, respect, safety, patience, empowerment, stability, and support in everyone's day-to-day life.

The person with LBD needs not only to feel loved, but also to feel safe and protected. What is often overlooked is that the person with LBD needs to feel empowered somewhere in life. The last vestige of that empowerment is often in an area no one is comfortable talking about—sexuality. The need for sex (especially for men), or at least the thought of it, seems to be present and does not always dissipate with time. You, as caregiver, barely have enough energy to get through a day, much less add sex to your agenda. Hugging, kissing, affectionate gestures, kind words are probably in your energy wheelhouse, and often using these loving tools will help calm the situation. As I mentioned, people hardly ever talk about this area, but it is more significant than is commonly acknowledged.

Someone with LBD picks up on mood and vibrations often with a heightened awareness. Love, dignity, and patience are the best gifts you can give someone with dementia of any kind. Your loved one may not always be able to express feelings or thoughts, but make no mistake, each person feels it all deeply. If you as caregiver are out of sorts, this will transfer. Phrases like "oh, you know you can do it, just try harder" or "just do it, you know how" are never helpful and can be harmful and hurtful. I am fond of saying: "If they could, they would, but they can't, so you have to work doubly hard at being patient and kind." And yes, *that's hard*, especially when you just want to scream.

By the way, I definitely recommend screaming or using a needed expletive when the going gets rough. Just be sure you can't be heard (screaming into a pillow works) and that your loved one doesn't see, hear, or feel your frustration. Give yourself permission to let it out, scream to your heart's content, breathe deeply, and then inhale the lovely scent of a lavender sachet or a scented bar of soap to calm down.

Support groups are invaluable resources. Your support group

members are also living in the world of LBD, and it's amazing how much they can help. You do learn more from those in the throes of this merciless journey than from almost any other resource. While it also helps to have truly good and understanding friends and relatives to help you navigate these rough waters, be aware to tread lightly as not everyone, no matter how close to you they may be, is up to the task of facing reality and then handling it. Try not to be disappointed by those you thought could handle it but can't.

Here are a few takeaways that I want to reemphasize:

- Love and dignity are the best gifts you can give anyone with LBD or any form of dementia.
- Making them feel safe, protected, and as much in control as they can be are important.
- If people with LBD could, they would . . . so please eliminate statements like "of course you know the answer, just try harder" or "oh, come on, you can do it."
- Arguing will just frustrate you and make your LBD loved one feel bad; if it's not a harmful situation, let your loved one have his or her way and don't be afraid to say "I'm sorry" even if it's not your fault.
- If your loved one is agitated, try to deflect the situation.
- Above all, be kind and gentle and patient.
- *And please know, all of this is easier said than done!*

General Information about Dementia

CaringKind is a New York City–based organization that defines itself as "NYC's leading expert on Alzheimer's and dementia caregiving," supporting individuals and families affected by dementia. In availing myself of their free classes, they provided the following general information, taken from my actual class notes for "Understanding Dementia," including Lewy body dementia and Alzheimer's disease:

- Dementia is associated with abnormal buildup of proteins in the brain creating problems.
- Cognitive problems include reasoning, judgment, behavior, recognizing consequences of actions; memory; ability to think.
- Motor skills, early hearing loss, vision, reading, and comprehension are affected.
- Early stage: still self-aware with ability to manage money; loss of initiative and motivation; aware of disease and able to share it; new things become a problem; less patience; stress exacerbates the system and makes things worse.
- Mid-stage: brain plays tricks; hallucinations/delusions; mood swings; motor problems; focus discomfort outward or everything becomes the other person's fault; confusion; important for caregiver not to argue or battle, to keep things upbeat and happy, to reduce stress; can't be left alone; there will be good and bad days; can't manage

their own money; beware of giving away money; need for supervision and direction; any drastic change is not good; be careful about what you as caregiver ask the person to do; with concern about loss of control comes issues of abandonment, frustration, safety; do things together.

- Late stage: probably need twenty-four-hour assistance; body affected; limited verbal ability; minimal recognition; difficulty eating; total incontinence.
- Be careful what you say, as the person understands on some level.
- Above all, maintain comfort and dignity.
- In general, don't force anything; careful not to display overt control; don't remind the person of the disease; only provide a choice when the answer doesn't matter, otherwise make the choice; validate the person.

And from the "Family Caregiver Workshop," the following proved invaluable:

- The person comes first, the disease comes second.
- Be aware of the person's depth perception and peripheral vision.
- Manage expectations: yours and theirs.
- Inappropriateness of person is compensation for what cannot be accessed.
- Stress is the enemy.
- Often the person has no filter or inhibitions.
- Person wants what they want when they want it.
- Fixed ideas are hard to get around.
- Behaviors need to be carefully managed.
- Try to see things from the person's perspective.
- The person cannot change; you have to change your expectations.

- The brain fills in blanks with delusions, ideas that are not real.
- The brain cannot connect because walls are being built.
- Important to know what makes a person feel safe; who do they ask for; what is their favorite thing.
- Important for the person to have a sense of purpose daily.
- As caregiver, be aware of your actions and reactions; be sure to take care of yourself—if you are not functioning, who will take care of your loved one?
- The person feels bad about being dependent.
- The disease is the driver, and it's important to show patience, flexibility, understanding.
- Eventually, managing and coping will require a team.
- Give people a daily plan to follow.
- Reminiscing is a good thing.
- Keep everything simple, slow, and supportive.
- Validation therapy: listen; really hear; agree with what's being said, even if you know it's not true, as it lessens stress. A simple "You are right! I am sorry" can go a long way; the person wants some control, so allow them to have it.
- Validate first, then redirect.
- Be in the moment.
- Express empathy.
- Helpful tools are music, art, poetry, and prayer.

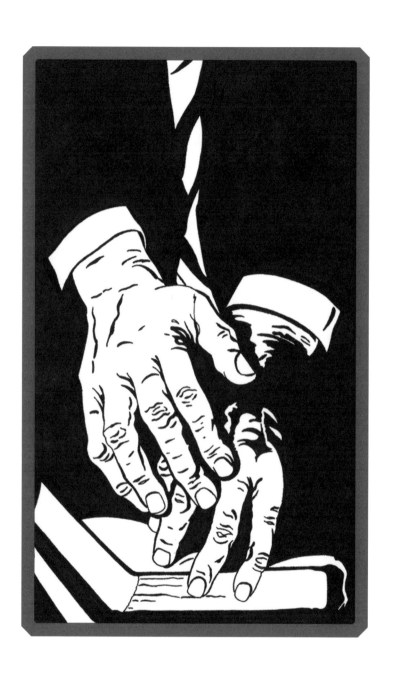

Helpful Resources

- **Lewy Body Dementia Resource Center:** www.lewybodyresourcecenter.org
  Helpline: 516-218-2026 or 833-LBD-LINE
- **CaringKind:** www.caringkindnyc.org
- **Lewy Body Society UK:** www.lewybody.org
- **Lewy Body Dementia Association:** www.lbda.org
- **Mayo Clinic:** www.mayoclinic.org
- **National Institute on Aging–National Institutes of Health:** www.nia.nih.gov
- **Michael J. Fox Foundation for Parkinson's Research:** www.michaeljfox.org

DISCLAIMER: While striving for accuracy is paramount, what I noted in my own research on Lewy body dementia is that sources are not always in agreement on the facts. In an effort to share core information about LBD in one consolidated place, the details about the disease throughout this book are assembled from a variety of sources: First and foremost from my real-life experience, plus information gleaned from caregiver support groups of the Lewy Body Dementia Resource Center and CaringKind, in addition to literature from the Mayo Clinic, National Institutes of Health, Lewy Body Society UK, among others.

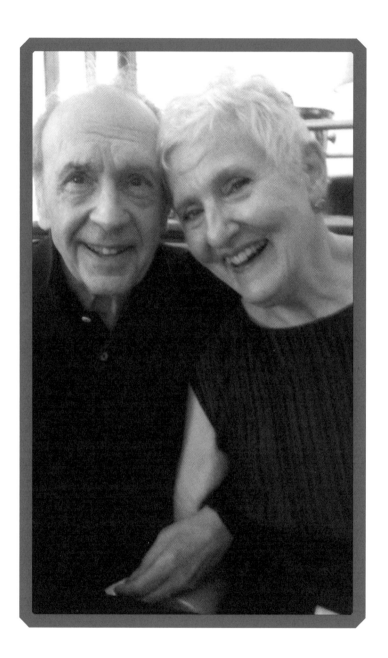

About the Author

MARY LOU FALCONE, a classical music strategist who founded M. L. Falcone, Public Relations in 1974 in New York City, helped guide and propel the careers of Van Cliburn, Renée Fleming, Gustavo Dudamel, Jean-Pierre Rampal, Nadja Salerno-Sonnenberg, Robert Shaw, Sir Georg Solti, Isaac Stern, James Taylor, Jaap van Zweden, and Eugenia Zukerman. She has also worked with the Birgit Nilsson Foundation, Carnegie Hall, Chicago Symphony, Los Angeles Philharmonic, New York Philharmonic, Philadelphia Orchestra, La Scala, Switzerland's Lucerne Festival, and the Vienna Philharmonic.

Born in Orange, New Jersey, she grew up in nearby rural Livingston. At age seventeen, she was accepted to the Curtis Institute of Music in Philadelphia where she studied voice. Upon graduating, she sang professionally for eight years with such organizations as NET Opera Theater and the Saint Paul Opera, soloed with orchestras, and sang oratorio. During this period, she was also a member of the faculty at the Baldwin School in Bryn Mawr, Pennsylvania, where she taught voice and general music for six years before chairing the music department, which she did for several years before forming her public relations company.

Additionally, she was on the faculty of the Juilliard School for twenty-two years and was a guest lecturer at Salzburg's Mozarteum University, Italy's Georg Solti Accademia, Manhattan School of Music, Mannes School of Music at the New School, and the Curtis Institute. She is currently on the board of the Lewy Body

Dementia Resource Center of New York, serves as a strategic advisor for DigiCARE Realized Inc., which focuses on modernizing care in the area of complex brain disease, and is an Executive Committee member of the Avery Fisher Artist Program at Lincoln Center. She has chaired both the Marilyn Horne Foundation and the Vatican/Rome-based Voices of Faith.

Mary Lou and illustrator Nicky Zann, devoted friends for forty-seven years, thirty-seven of which they were also a couple, were married three years before Nicky passed away in 2020.

For more information, please visit: www.MaryLouFalcone.com.

About the Illustrator

NICHOLAS "NICKY" ZANN (1943–2020) was a popular 1950s rock 'n' roll musician and a world-renowned cartoonist and illustrator for such publications as *Newsweek*, the *New York Times*, numerous comics, and mystery book covers. Nicky's drawings from *The Answer Deck*, a fortune-telling card game he created and designed, which sold 100,000 copies, are featured throughout this book.

As a musician, Nicky toured internationally from 1957 to 1965, often appearing on the same shows as Jerry Lee Lewis, Patsy Cline, and Johnny Cash. In 1965, inspired by a commission for ABC's *Les Crane Show*, he turned his sights to art, continuing his studies at the School of Visual Arts, guided by Jack Potter and Burne Hogarth. His artwork was singled out several times by Johnny Carson on NBC's *Tonight Show*, and in 1990, MTV aired a special premier edition of profiles on Karl Lagerfeld, Andy Warhol, and Nicky Zann.

In 1970, he created "Love Comic," which was first exhibited in London's Victoria and Albert Museum in 1974. His work remains part of the museum's permanent pop art collection and, according to the museum, was said to inspire the work of Roy Lichtenstein. In the late 1980s, Nicky added abstract figurative oil paintings to his portfolio, including a seven-foot theatrical panel commissioned to accompany Pulitzer Prize–winning composer John Harbison's chamber music piece *November 19, 1828* (the day Schubert died), which debuted at New York's Merkin Concert